THE PROTEIN EXPRESS DIET

**A NEW STRATEGY FOR
RAPID WEIGHT LOSS WITH A SIMPLIFIED
LOW-CARB, HIGH PROTEIN DIET**

by M. R. Ford

OSK Publishing

CONTENTS

INTRODUCTION

<u>IMPORTANT NOTE</u>: NONE OF THE INFORMATION IN THIS BOOK CONSTITUTES MEDICAL ADVICE. BEFORE UNDERTAKING ANY DIET OR EXERCISE PROGRAM, BE SURE TO CONSULT WITH YOUR DOCTOR, ESPECIALLY IF YOU HAVE ANY KNOWN HEALTH ISSUES.

This is not a book written by some preternaturally thin person who offers to instruct the rest of us in the art of weight loss and maintenance. I have a very strong genetic predisposition to pack on the pounds. I was a consistently overweight child and teenager who later soared well into the obesity range in early adulthood.

When it comes to losing weight and keeping it off, I am one of the tough cases. I have written this book because I believe the things that work for me will work for you as well. The weight loss strategy described in these pages grew out of my personal experience as I have struggled with a lifelong natural tendency to put on weight. The results speak for themselves: I was able to lose a total of 70 pounds, going from a weight of nearly 210 pounds to about 140. While on the diet, I lost an average of 8-15 pounds per month, and I have been able to maintain my weight for the last twenty years— although doing so sometimes presented a challenge, and as a result, I developed a very specific and effective strategy for dealing with inevitable tendency to regain weight (or "yo-yo").

I developed this protein-intensive, low-carbohydrate diet independently—primarily on the basis of self-experimentation and research—long before I had heard of Dr. Dukan's program, which has now brought a great deal of attention to diets of this type. The primary difference between my Protein Express Diet and other diets is that I have placed a very strong emphasis on convenience, quick preparation and affordability. I started my weight loss program as a single guy who then (and now) hates to cook or spend time preparing food. I had an "on the run" lifestyle, and prior to beginning my diet ate most of my meals out—often resorting to poor choices such as fast food. My goal was to create a diet that worked with that lifestyle, was highly affordable and did not require extensive food preparation. Over the years, I have constantly refined and improved my weight loss strategy by incorporating the latest research and innovations in the science of nutrition.

As a result, the diet described here will be a good match for those who do not enjoy cooking. It will also work well for busy families. In many cases there is simply not time (or energy) to prepare two completely different meals on a regular basis. The Protein Express Diet offers a solution.

The Protein Express Diet can be used independently, or it can be integrated into the Dukan or Atkins diet—or into virtually any low-carb or low-fat diet. In the chapters that follow I will lay out a very simple, five step plan that will result in rapid and consistent weight loss. This is the plan that worked for me, and I am confident that it will work for you.

On the other hand, if you are already familiar with an established diet such as Dukan, Atkins or South Beach and prefer to follow the rules advocated by these diets, then you can use the techniques in this book to make meal preparation faster, easier and more affordable while adding high quality protein to your diet. The meals described here, will fit perfectly into the Dukan/Atkins/South Beach system and offer an alternative when you simply don't have time for extensive food preparation.

In addition to the diet, this book also includes information on exercise, including a innovative high intensity walking technique that will allow you to dramatically increase the number calories you burn while walking. Also covered, is a quick and simple weight training program to help you maintain muscle mass while you lose weight. The exercise techniques are completely optional. The diet will work by itself, and you can feel free to mix and match the diet, walking and weight training routines based on your preferences and objectives.

The book is divided into four chapters:

Chapter 1: Overview of Macronutrients and The Importance of Protein

- Explains the role of the macronutrients: carbohydrates, fat and protein. Also covers the role of the hormone insulin, and explains the critical role of protein.
- Includes an overview of low-carbohydrate, protein-intensive diets (including the Dukan and Atkins diets), the advantages of these diets, and why they work.

Chapter 2: The Protein Express Diet

- Gives specific instructions for creating highly nutritious, affordable and easy to prepare protein-intensive meals.
- Covers a simple 5-step plan for using the Protein Express Diet to achieve rapid weight loss—and then keep the weight off forever.
- Alternatively, shows how to use the Protein Express Diet in conjunction with the Dukan or Atkins diets, or with virtually any other diet.
- Covers the Protein Express Diet for vegans or vegetarians.
- Offers suggestions for breaking a fast food and snack habit.
- Provides a specific strategy for "drawing a line in the sand" regarding weight gain once you get into the maintenance phase of your diet, and provides a highly effective and proven technique for taking immediate action so you can stop yo-yo weight gain in its tracks.

Chapter 3: Exercise

- Introduces walking as an exercise and explains why it is the most effective choice for a on-going exercise plan that you are likely to stick with over time.

- Offers specific tips for making walking more enjoyable and tools to help select an outdoor route.
- Describes an innovative way to "turbo charge" your walking so that you can burn more fat and develop more mus-

cle without the need to invest more time. This technique does not require any extra equipment or expense and will work with either outdoor or treadmill walking.

- Offers tips on developing a very simple and very fast (as little as 10 minutes per workout) plan for using weight training to retain muscle mass during weight loss and build muscle and strength over the long term.

- Includes the basic facts—supported by real research— that you need to know in order to develop quick and easy workouts that you are more likely to stick with. This section is NOT geared toward bodybuilding or people who want highly intensive training, but rather those who want to stay fit with the absolute minimum investment of time and energy.

Chapter 4: Thermal Weight Loss Techniques

- This chapter provides an overview of some relatively new ideas on the impact of temperature on weight loss.

My objective in writing this book is to present the information, tips and tricks that I have accumulated in my twenty-year successful battle with my natural, genetic tendency to be overweight. I have not set out to write a long book, but rather the most concise and effective presentation possible. At a price of $2.99—less than the average drink at Starbucks—I believe it offers an extraordinary value for those who want a simple and effective weight loss strategy that really works. If you make a commitment to employ the strategies and techniques explained here, I believe that this book could very well change your life.

A CONCISE OVERVIEW OF THE MACRONUTRIENTS: CARBOHYDRATES, FAT AND PROTEIN

All the food we eat can be broken down into three basic categories known as macronutrients: carbohydrates (starches and sugars), fats and protein. The average diet is heavily skewed toward carbohydrates. Carbohydrates are the easiest and simplest type of food to digest and turn into energy.

Foods like pasta, rice, bread, cake, candy, beer and sugar-laden soft drinks all consist primarily of extremely energy-dense carbohydrate. Foods of this type are digested rapidly and efficiently and are broken down into glucose—a simple sugar that provides energy to your cells. If the amount of energy taken in (measured in calories) exceeds what you are expending through physical exercise and normal metabolism, that additional energy will be stored as fat. The hormone insulin plays a critical role in determining the likelihood that the energy you consume will end up being stored as fat. We'll look at how insulin works in the next section.

Fats are also an important source of energy; however, your body needs to do somewhat more work to digest them. While carbohydrates begin to be broken down in your mouth and stomach, digestion of fat occurs in the small intestine and requires the cooperation of both the liver and the pancreas to provide the necessary enzymes. Fats are broken down into components called fatty acids, which can then be used by your body as fuel.

For the most part, fatty acids and carbohydrates (glucose) can act as interchangeable energy sources for your body. There is one very important exception, however: your brain cannot use fatty acids as an energy source. This is because fatty acids are unable to cross the blood-brain barrier—a protective mechanism that keeps pathogens like bacteria as well as large, complex molecules like fatty acids from being able to invade your nervous system from your blood stream.

If you restrict yourself to a low-carbohydrate diet, you will soon exhaust the glucose that normally powers your brain function. At this point, your body will have to produce a substitute energy source that is capable of crossing the blood-brain barrier. This substitute energy source consists of what are called ketone bodies. These are smaller, energy-laden molecules that are able to cross into the brain from the blood stream.

Ketone bodies are produced in the liver from fatty acids. When your body has an elevated level of ketone bodies you are said to be in a state of ketosis. In other words, you are powering your body on the basis of fat (hopefully, including your body's stored fat), rather than carbohydrates. As your body burns the ketone bodies as fuel, it produces the chemical acetone as a byproduct. Acetone is the solvent that is used in products like nail polish remover. This waste acetone gets expelled in your urine and in your breath. As a result, Ketosis often produces a distinctive breath odor.

The third type of of food—protein—fulfills a unique role. Proteins are quite literally the primary building blocks that constitute nearly all the structures of the your body, with the exception of bones and fat. In addition to structural tissue like muscle, skin and internal organs, the essential chemicals that your body depends on—such as digestive enzymes—likewise consist of protein molecules.

Proteins are very large and complex molecules that are constructed by stringing together smaller molecules called amino acids. There are twenty different amino acids, but they can be combined in almost limitless number of different ways to create all the different proteins that make up your body. Your genetic code (DNA) is actually a type of recipe for constructing proteins from amino acid building blocks.

Your body is constantly tearing down protein structures (including muscle and other components of your body) and then reconstructing them. This is a normal process that occurs regardless of whether or not you are attempting to lose weight and is called "protein turnover." To support this process, your body will maintain a fairly constant supply of amino acid building blocks in your blood stream. These amino acids may come from food that you digest and/or from structures that are constantly being broken down.

If the amount of protein you ingest is insufficient, then your body will rely primarily on cannibalizing muscle tissue and other structures to maintain the necessary supply of amino acids in your blood stream. In other words, the lean tissue in your body will enter a so-called catabolic state, where your body essentially begins to feed on itself. This is the reason that most people who go on diets tend to lose significant muscle as well as fat.

While the amino acids that make up protein are essential building blocks for your body's tissues, they can also be broken down and used to produce energy. As with fat, the process for turning protein into energy is more complex and less efficient than is the case with carbohydrates. Amino acids are broken down into other simpler molecules which can then be used to produce the glucose your cells require as an energy source. This happens in your liver, using a chemical process called deamination. Just as the chemical reaction that turns fatty acids into ketone bodies produces acetone as a waste product, deamination of amino acids produces ammonia—a toxic chemical that must be further processed in your kidneys before being expelled in your urine.

As someone who is attempting to lose fat, you would of course strongly prefer that your body use all the protein you ingest to maintain your muscle and other lean structures, while relying solely on your stored fat as an energy source. Unfortunately, that is not the way things work, and there really is no way to precisely control (or even measure) what percentage of the protein you eat will be used as an energy source rather than as building material for your body.

There is important evidence to suggest, however, that consuming a relatively higher percentage of protein in your diet will at least help minimize the amount of lean body cannibalization that will occur when you attempt to lose weight. Scientists and medical doctors have studied the effects of extreme (starvation-level) diets and found that higher protein intake does help preserve lean tissue. For example, here is what the medical textbook Modern Nutrition in Health and Disease has to say on the subject:

10

> ...the major influence on protein turnover is pro-
> tein intake itself. Thus, very low energy (500 cal-
> ories/day) reducing diets that include generous
> amounts of high quality protein maintain protein
> turnover, whereas fasting or low-energy diets
> low in good-quality protein reduce it. (p. 738)

In other words, any time you attempt to lose weight by restricting your food intake, there are good reasons to make sure that protein makes up a significantly higher than normal percentage of the food you are eating. Doing so should help to prevent your protein turnover from entering a catabolic state where you lose significant lean tissue.

The minimum protein intake recommended by the U.S. government is about 0.8 grams per kilogram (or 0.36 grams per pound) of body weight. For a typical, non-dieting person who consumes about 2000 calories per day, this works out to about 50-60 grams of protein each day. Nearly anyone who eats a normal Western diet will have little trouble taking in sufficient protein to meet this guideline. Again, that number is for someone who is eating a balanced diet and is satisfied with maintaining his or her current weight. As we've seen, if you want to lose fat by modifying or restricting your food intake, you should consume significantly more protein than the guidelines specify. That is one of the primary advantages of protein-intensive diets like the Protein Express Diet or the Dukan Diet.

While increasing your protein intake will hopefully help minimize the amount of lean tissue that is lost when you attempt to lose fat, there is no guarantee that muscle loss can be prevented entirely. Nearly everyone who goes on a diet in an attempt to lose

11

fat also loses muscle. In order to prevent this, it is strongly recommended that you combine higher protein intake with some form of weight training or resistance exercise. Just as a business starved for revenue will be likely to first lay off non-essential employees, your body is likely to cannibalize muscles that are not being used, and this is a significant danger if you maintain a sedentary lifestyle while dieting. For this reason, this book contains a brief section on how to get the most out of very brief weight training sessions. The point of this is to trick your body into believing that your muscles are essential for your survival; this will greatly reduce any lean tissue loss, and may even make it possible for you to gain muscle while on your diet.

KEY POINTS ABOUT MACRONUTRIENTS

Here's a brief summary of the important things to keep in mind about macronutrients:

- Carbohydrates are by far the easiest to digest and turn into energy. Excess energy will rapidly be stored as fat.

- Fats and proteins are more difficult to digest. Breaking them down requires the cooperation of organs such as the liver and pancreas, and the digestive process uses more energy (calories).

- Protein fulfills a unique dual role: it provides the essential amino acid building blocks that are used to maintain nearly all your body's structural tissue and functional chemicals. Proteins can also be converted to energy, and then stored as fat if excess amounts are consumed.

- Consuming a higher protein diet while attempting to lose weight has been demonstrated to help minimize loss of lean tissue. To further reduce the risk of losing muscle, some form of weight-bearing or resistance exercise is strongly recommended.

HOW PROTEINS ARE CONSTRUCTED AND BROKEN DOWN - A VIDEO SIMULATION

To get an idea of how protein molecules are built from amino acids and then broken down by your cells, watch this short ABC News special that features an amazing video simulation "Inner Life of a Cell" created by a Harvard scientist:

YouTube:
http://www.youtube.com/watch?v=GVqJdAqTD4Q&feature=related

Tip: Rather than typing in the URL above, just search YouTube for "inner life of a cell".

HOW INSULIN CAUSES YOUR BODY TO STORE FAT

Whenever you consume carbohydrates, your pancreas will release the hormone insulin into your bloodstream. The primary purpose of insulin is to force your liver, muscle and fat cells to remove glucose from your blood stream; this prevents the glucose level in your blood from reaching toxic levels. Once your body's energy needs have been fulfilled, any excess glucose is converted by your cells into fatty acids that circulate in your blood stream.

Insulin causes your fat cells to act like "roach motels" for fatty acids: fatty acids can enter your fat cells where they are linked up and stored as more complex molecules called triglycerides; however, they cannot exit your fat cells and enter your bloodstream. In other words, insulin shuts down the use of fat as fuel for your body and instead shifts you into fat storage mode. Obviously, this is a very undesirable state for anyone who wants to lose fat!

Research shows that insulin release begins immediately—in fact, in can occur before you even begin eat, just as a result of thinking about an upcoming meal. As you eat more carbohydrates—and in particular—simple, easily digested sugars and starches, the level of insulin in your blood will increase rapidly. In his book *Why We Get Fat: And What to Do About It*, Gary Taubes makes a compelling argument that the "calories in/calories out" calculation that underlies most traditional diets is destined to fail in large measure because it ignores the role that insulin plays in fat storage.

Numerous scientific studies on animals have shown that the accumulation of fat is governed by hormonal factors—and occurs regardless of whether or not animals are allowed to overeat. For example, squirrels naturally grow fatter in order to support hibernation through the winter. Scientists have found that even if the squirrels' diets are restricted, they still gain weight. Similar results have been found by manipulating animals in ways that increases the amount of insulin in their blood: weight gain invariably occurs even if the animals do not eat more food.

The bottom line is that anyone who wants to lose fat—or, in other words, burn fat as fuel rather than store it—has to be very concerned about avoiding high levels of insulin in their blood stream. People who follow a traditional low-fat diet, often make the mistake of skewing their food intake even more in the direction of carbohydrates. This is especially a problem if you rely on packaged foods that are labeled as "low in fat." Very often, these products are loaded with exactly the refined sugars and starches that are most likely to result in the increased insulin levels that will switch your metabolism into fat storage mode.

The best way to keep your insulin level under control is to minimize your consumption of carbohydrates, and in particular the simple sugars and starches often found in snacks, desserts, sweet beverages and processed foods. These foods result in a rapid increase in the glucose levels in your blood and, in turn, that will cause large amounts of insulin to be released.

THE GLYCEMIC INDEX—USE WITH CAUTION!

In order to measure the impact of a particular food on blood sugar levels (and therefore on insulin), scientists have developed a measure called the glycemic index. The higher the glycemic index, the faster your blood glucose will increase after eating that food. Here are a few example glycemic index values:

Doughnut: 76

White Bread: 71

Table Sugar: 65

Mango: 56

Banana: 54

Whole Grain Bread: 50

Snickers Bar: 40

Apple: 38

Broccoli: 15

The general idea behind the glycemic index is, of course, that you should avoid foods with a high index and select those with a lower index. However, if you look at the list above you you can see some fairly obvious problems with giving too much weight to this index. Does anyone really believe that eating a Snickers bar is roughly equivalent to eating an apple—and more healthy than eating a banana? The reality is that the glycemic index says nothing about the amount of carbohydrate (and calories) in a particular food. A snack food like a Snickers bar has a lower index primarily because it contains peanuts along with all the sugar. That does result in a lower average glycemic index, but it obviously does not change the fact that the sugar is present and will cause your insulin level to increase and your body to store fat.

My personal approach is to use the glycemic index only as a way to pick out those basic foods that have a very low score. The best strategy is to pick foods that have a low glycemic index and are also low in calories. For example, non-starchy vegetables like broccoli and spinach have an index of only 15 as well as a very low calorie count. That, together with the known health benefits of these vegetables makes them an excellent choice with any meal.

If you want to limit insulin levels and turn your body's fat storage switch to the off position—and engage the fat burning process—the best way is to simply avoid eating carbohydrates, with the exception of those healthy vegetables that have very little starch or sugar, very few calories and a low glycemic index. At all costs, you must avoid eating processed sugary foods and beverages.

LOW CARBOHYDRATE DIETS, HOW THEY WORK AND DIFFERENT APPROACHES

THE ATKINS DIET

The original low carbohydrate diet was introduced by Dr. Robert Atkins in 1972. Dr. Atkins latest book, *Atkins New Diet Revolution*, lays out the details of his approach.

The Atkins diet was highly controversial and was for many years opposed by organizations such as the American Heart Association. This was primarily because the Atkins diet calls for increased intake of protein and fat—and does not limit the consumption of the saturated fats that have been associated with illnesses such as heart disease. In more recent years, low-carbohydrate diets have gained more acceptance, but many experts remain opposed to consuming saturated fat in significant amounts.

Dr. Atkins primary rationale for his diet is that the digestion and metabolism of protein and fat is much less efficient than is the case with carbohydrates. While a person a may consume the same number of calories in the form of fat/protein or carbohydrate, the net impact from the fat or protein will be significantly lower because it takes more energy to digest those food types.

The initial or "induction" phase of the Atkins diet is highly restrictive and allows only 20 grams of carbohydrate per day. The purpose of this restriction is to force your body into a state of ketosis—where fat is broken down and used to power your brain and other organs.

The Atkins diet has been enormously popular, with tens of millions of people trying the diet. Recent research has shown that low carbohydrate diets can be more effective than low fat diets—at least in the short term. However, there is significant controversy over how the diets really work. Some experts think that eating more protein and fat is simply more filling, and therefore, people tend to consume fewer calories. Others give more credence to Dr. Atkins argument that the diet offers an on-going metabolic advantage since proteins and fats require more energy to digest. As we saw in the previous section, the control of your body's insulin levels is also an important argument in favor of low carb diets.

THE DUKAN DIET

The low carbohydrate movement started by Dr. Atkins has evolved over time, and there are now a number of different diets with varying strategies and philosophies. Dr. Pierre Dukan's diet has been popular in France for many years, and was recently introduced in the United States via his book, *The Dukan Diet*. The key difference with the Dukan diet is that it strongly emphasizes the consumption of lean protein rather than fat.

Dukan argues that only about 50% of foods like meat or fish are assimilated by the body; the rest is tissue that cannot be digested and goes to waste. In other words, protein foods are more filling because a larger quantity of food results in fewer calories actually becoming available to the body. This is somewhat similar to eating high-fiber vegetables—except that most people find protein dishes more satisfying.

Dukan also believes that humans have a metabolism that works best with a ratio for food types of 5 parts carbohydrate to 3 parts fat to 2 parts protein. In other words, when foods are consumed according to this natural 5-3-2 ratio, digestion and metabolism will be most efficient, and weight gain may result. Dukan suggests that a weight loss diet should seek to upset this ratio by focusing exclusively on one food type. The only practical choice for doing that is protein, since (as we saw earlier) amino acid building blocks are essential for maintaining your body's structural elements.

PROTEIN VS FAT

The approach I lay out in this book is much closer to the Dukan than the Atkins diet. The primary reason is that I believe there is very strong evidence to suggest that consuming large amounts of fat—and especially saturated fat—is a very bad idea. Consider, for example, what cardiologist Arthur Agaston says in his book, *The South Beach Diet*:

> The major problem I have with the Atkins Diet is the liberal intake of saturated fats. There is evidence now that immediately following a meal of saturated fats, there is dysfunction in the arteries, including those that supply the heart muscle with blood. As a result, the lining of the ar-

teries (the endothelium) is predisposed to constriction and clotting. Imagine: Under the right (or rather, wrong) circumstances, eating a meal that's high in saturated fat can trigger a heart attack! (page 21-22)

While some some advocates of low carbohydrate diets, including Dr. Atkins, have pushed back against the conventional belief that excessive intake of saturated fat is unhealthy, I continue to think there are good reasons to limit the total amount of fat, and in particular saturated fat in your diet. There is also compelling evidence that some types of fat, especially monounsaturated fats like olive oil, and to a somewhat lesser extent, polyunsaturated vegetable oils like corn oil, actually provide important health benefits, such as regulation of cholesterol levels. Therefore, the strategy I advocate in this book is to consume a protein-intensive, low carbohydrate diet with moderate fat intake. Saturated fat should be limited (but not eliminated), and to the extent possible, the fat you consume should be of the healthy monounsaturated variety.

PALEO DIETS

A more recent, and very popular, argument in favor of a low carbohydrate diet is the "paleo" movement. The main idea is that humans are biologically designed to live and eat as hunter-gathers. Paleo diets are named after the paleolithic period, which covers the time from when human beings first appeared up until roughly ten thousand years ago. During this prehistoric period, people would have survived primarily by hunting and fishing, and by gathering naturally available plant-based foods. Technology would have been limited to simple stone tools and spears, and the advent of agriculture remained thousands of years in the future.

Without agricultural technology, people simply would have not had access to the high energy content carbohydrates that make up the bulk of the modern diet. Bread, rice and other foods that rely on harvesting large amounts of grain would have been unknown. Meat and fish would likely have been a primary, year-round source of food, while plant foods would have been highly seasonal and limited to what could be found nearby. The wild animals hunted and eaten would have certainly have been much more lean than the domesticated, typically grain-fed, cattle that we eat today. One of the best books on paleo-style diets is *The New Evolution Diet*, by Arthur De Vany, who has followed the diet for over twenty-five years.

INTRODUCING THE PROTEIN EXPRESS DIET

The key component of the Protein Express Diet is high quality protein powder formulated from either whey (a byproduct of cheese production) or soy. Protein powders offer the highest concentration of high quality protein available in any food, and they are also more affordable, per gram of protein, than most meat, fish or dairy products.

Protein powders are primarily marketed to bodybuilders and athletes. These people are generally not at all interested in losing weight. Instead they eat generously and then supplement their diets with protein powder—sometimes in extreme amounts—in order to support muscle growth. Bodybuilders typically spend hours each week in the gym lifting weights, and then consume huge amounts of protein in the hope of packing on ever more muscle.

The irony is that research has shown that such extreme protein consumption is probably not necessary for already fit people on non-restrictive diets who want to add muscle. While these individuals may require somewhat more protein, their normal diets probably already provide enough to support muscle growth. The fact is that protein powders may actually be more useful for people who are primarily interested in losing fat. This is because they offer a

very low-carbohydrate—and low calorie—way to add lots of protein to your diet and thus help avoid losing muscle and other lean
tissue as you lose fat.

Later in this book, I will offer a specific and easy to follow plan for
using protein powder in conjunction with other protein-based
foods to create a low-carb diet that should consistently result in a
weight loss of about 2-4 pounds per week for most people. Protein
powder will also fit neatly into either the Dukan or Atkins diet—
adding variety and making the diets more affordable.

I will show you exactly how to mix protein drinks or shakes so that
you maximize protein while minimizing carbohydrate and fat. I'll
even show you how to do that while still including many of the
dietary benefits of important vegetables like spinach and broccoli
as well as the fiber that is important for healthy digestion. And you
can do all that without cooking and at a cost that is typically far
less per meal than stopping for fast food. The time it takes to prepare a protein powder-based meal is far less than waiting in line at
McDonald's—and the nutritional quality of the meal is immeasur-
ably superior.

There are a number of important ways you can use protein powder-based meals:

- You can use a protein drink or shake as a complete meal
  replacement on a regular basis. Breakfast is an ideal
  choice because it saves you time, and ensures a fast and
  easy high protein meal in a situation where many people
  people make the mistake of consuming too many carbohydrates and too little protein.

- You can use protein shakes in situations where you are in a rush and might typically fall back on unwise choices like fast food or vending machines. You can easily keep the ingredients you need for a protein powder meal in the trunk of your car or in your desk at work—so they are always available. If you are hungry and need an especially filling meal, I'll show you how to thicken the drink to make it more satisfying without adding fat, carbohydrates or calories. In any case, you will find that these meals are more satisfying that you might expect because of the high protein content.

- Protein drinks and desserts can be used to add variety to meals that consist primarily of meat, fish and other protein sources (as for example recommended by the Dukan diet). Rather than sitting down to a large meal consisting entirely of meat, you will be able to have a meat dish followed by a protein drink or dessert. This also makes your meal more affordable, because you can eat less meat— and the lower overall cost may make it possible for you to select better quality meat or fish.

- If you have family members who are not sharing your diet, protein drinks will allow you to avoid cooking two separate meals. You can simply eat a normal helping of the protein portion of your family's meal while skipping the carbohydrates. You can then augment your own meal with a protein drink or dessert.

- Because protein drinks are sweet and typically have flavours like chocolate or vanilla, your body will perceive them as primarily carbohydrates, even though they are almost entirely protein. This will you control carb-carving

25

and greatly reduce the feeling that you are missing out by keeping to a high protein/low carbohydrate diet.

FOOD SAFETY AND NUTRITION

One obvious question you may have is whether or not a diet that incorporates significant amounts of protein powder is nutritious or advisable. Isn't it always better to consume whole foods as opposed to powders?

If we were talking about fruits and vegetables, then the answer would almost certainly be YES. However, with meat and fish the answer is more complex. The reality is that if you are going to pursue a low carbohydrate/high protein diet, you will necessarily be consuming meat and fish in relatively high quantities. And these foods have a number of safety issues associated with them.

With vegetables, you have the option of purchasing organic products from a local farmer's market or perhaps even growing your own produce in your garden. With meat and fish, you have far less control over where your food is coming from and how it is processed.

As an example, The Dukan diet recommends both tilapia, a fish that is high in protein and low in fat, and shrimp. Both of these foods are allowed options in the Dukan diet's "attack phase" where you consume only protein, and you are allowed to eat as much as you like.

That sounds great—unless you happen to have read the recent book Death by China by Peter W. Navarro and Greg Autry. It turns out that China dominates the market for both tilapia and shrimp. Here's what the authors have to say about how these products are produced in Chinese fish farms:

> Today China is the world's leading source of farm-raised fish and dominates the markets for catfish, tilapia, shrimp and eel....Along the Yangtze [river]'s route, booming cities such as Chengdu and Chongquinq dump billions of tons of mostly untreated human, animal, and industrial waste directly into the river. This toxic mess is then given some considerable time to ferment and stew as it collects in the reservoir behind the gigantic Three Gorges Dam.

> ...remember that it is precisely this Yangtze stew...that fills the export-focused fish farms on China's East Coast. Of course, because Chinese eels, fish and shrimp are raised in such toxic conditions, the creatures suffer from all manner of infections and parasites....To treat these conditions, China's fish farmers routinely pump all manner of banned antibiotics, antifungals, antivirals, and dyes into their polluted waters. These toxic substances, which are inevitably absorbed into the creatures' flesh, range from malachite green, choloramphenicol, and flouroquinolones to nitrofurans, contraceptive drugs, and gentian violet; and they do everything from cause cancer and trigger rare diseases like aplastic anemia to degrade the human body's ability to use antibiotics to cure infections. (pp. 25-26)

Clearly, while shrimp and tilapia may be "whole" foods, they are not necessarily something you want to consume in large quantities! Of course, you can select wild, rather than farmed, fish but this will be significantly more expensive, and in the case of tilapia, may be higher in mercury.

Perhaps you prefer to avoid seafood from China and eat more American beef. Lean cuts of beef are another item recommended for the attack phase of the Dukan diet.

The book Fast Food Nation by Eric Schlosser (also a movie) tells the story of the U.S. meatpacking industry and how it has come to be completely dominated by the needs of the fast food industry. Workers are low-paid, unskilled and often do not speak English. The production line moves at an astonishingly fast rate—so that workers are typically exhausted and errors are common. Workers look forward to the days when the beef is to be exported to the European Union (including Dr. Dukan's home country of France), because the production line must then be slowed to approximately half its normal rate in order to insure safety and quality. However, as soon as the beef is destined for the U.S. domestic market, the line goes back to full speed.

The meat packing and processing industry has enormous influence over regulators and is often able to limit the authority of federal safety inspectors. At one point, the industry actually managed to have inspectors removed entirely, shifting responsibility for inspections to the industry itself. Fast Food Nation tells how that worked out:

> ....visibly diseased animals—cattle infected with measles and tapeworms, covered with abscesses—were being slaugh-

tered. Poorly trained company inspectors were allowing the shipment of beef contaminated with fecal material, hair, insects, metal shavings, urine and vomit. (p. 207)

Fortunately, the government inspectors are now back on the job, but the ability of regulators to insure quality or force companies to recall contaminated products continues to be very limited.

By now you may feel that protein powder does not seem so bad after all! My point is not to trash all meat and fish products, but rather to point out that a reflexive preference for whole foods does not necessarily make sense. Protein powder is generally a very safe and nutritious component for your diet.

In addition, protein powder is very affordable, and that may help you to make better choices with the meat and fish products you consume. Supplementing a protein-intensive dinner with a relatively inexpensive protein powder-based dessert may allow you to spend more money on the main dish. Rather that consume large amounts of cheap meat or fish, select the non-farmed (wild) fish and choose grass-fed beef or the organic, free range chicken. These choices are harder to find, and they may cost significantly more. But by eating a little less meat, and following it with a protein drink, you not only add variety to your meal, you can also greatly enhance the quality and safety of your primary protein dishes.

It goes without saying that when selecting protein powders it is also important to take care. While I am aware of no case in which a reputable brand of commercial protein powder has been shown to be intentionally adulterated, there have been cases where other products produced in China have had toxic chemicals like melamine added in place of protein. This famously led to the deaths of pets in the United States in cases where dog and cat food was adulterated, and even more tragically to the death of infants in China when baby formula was manipulated.

There has been documentation of other forms of contamination for protein powder in a few cases. The July, 2010 issue of Consumer Reports found that a few brands of protein power—if consumed in very large amounts—had unsafe levels of heavy metals, such as cadmium. Protein powder—or for that matter anything you will be consuming in significant quantities—is clearly not something you want to pick up at a flea market or the dollar store. Buy only known brands from reputable retailers. In the next section, I will tell you what to look for in protein powders and also recommend the specific brands that I use myself. I also strongly recommend that you follow the general safety guidelines below.

USING PROTEIN POWDER SUPPLEMENTS SAFELY

- The Protein Express Diet (and the use of protein powder supplements) is **NOT for you if**: You are pregnant (or think you might be), if you are under age 18, or if you have known health issues, in particular problems with your kidneys. If you have any doubts, be certain to consult your physician.
- Never replace more than two meals per day with protein drinks, and never consume more than six servings of protein powder (about 150 grams of protein) in any single day.

- I suggest mixing roughly equal portions of two types of protein powder (soy and whey) from two different manufacturers; this will help insure that you are not consuming large amounts of product from any one source in the unlikely event that some type of contamination should occur.
- If you use a brand of protein powder not specifically recommended here, I suggest checking the July, 2010 issue of Consumer Reports to make sure your brand is not on the problem list. You should be able to find this in your local library.

WHEY VS. SOY PROTEIN

There are a variety of different types of protein power available. However, the two types that offer the highest quality protein at the lowest cost are whey and soy. Whey is a liquid that is left over when milk is processed into cheese. To produce whey protein powder, the liquid whey is further processed to isolate the protein from fat and other substances. Soy protein powder is produced by processing soybeans so that the protein is isolated from other substances.

Both whey and soy are high quality "complete" proteins. As I mentioned earlier, there are twenty types of amino acid building blocks that make up protein. Of these twenty, nine are not able to be synthesized from other components by your body—they are called "essential" because they must be consumed in food. Proteins that contain all nine of these essential amino acids are called "complete." Nearly all foods that offer complete proteins are animal based: meat, fish, and dairy products. Soy is the only stand-alone plant-based complete protein. It's possible to get all the essential amino acids from other plants, but you have to mix and match different grains or vegetables in order to create complete protein.

Among some athletes and bodybuilders, there has traditionally been a strong bias for whey protein as opposed to soy. In part, this is because soy protein contains phytoestrogens—chemicals that are closely related to the female hormone estrogen. This has led to some concern that soy protein might in some way inhibit testosterone production and thereby limit muscle growth. However, recent studies have shown that that soy protein is effective in supporting muscle growth, and a number of successful vegetarian bodybuilders have used soy protein exclusively. In addition, the phytoestrogens in soy may have important health benefits. Some researchers believe that consumption of soy-based foods results in a lower risk for breast and prostate cancer; however, the evidence is not yet conclusive.

Another difference between whey and soy is the degree of bioavailability (BV) for the protein. Bioavailability is a measure of the extent to which a nutrient becomes available to your tissues after being fully digested. Whey protein is considered to be the "gold standard" of bioavailability with a value of 104. Soy, by contrast, has a value of about 74.

The table below shows the bioavailability (BV) for several types of protein:

Whey	104
Egg	100
Milk	91
Beef	80
Fish	79
Chicken	77
Soy	74

You can see from the table above why bodybuilders and others who are focused on consuming extreme amounts of protein may prefer whey. However, as someone who is striving to lose weight a high BV is probably less important, and may even be an advantage if you consume excessive amounts. My personal preference is to use both whey and soy protein. I like to mix the two types together in order to gain the benefits of both. However, if you have a strong preference for one or the other, or if there is a substantial differ-ence in cost, it is fine to use one type exclusively. Obviously, if you are a vegetarian or vegan, then soy protein is your only option.

BEYOND PROTEIN: GREENS AND FIBER

In addition to protein powder, I strongly recommend that you use one of the many available "green supplement" products in the drinks you create for the Protein Express Diet. These products contain extracts of a variety of important vegetables and sometimes fruits.

The primary reason for including green supplement powder is not to provide vitamins. The list of standard vitamins and minerals that you require on a daily basis is well known, and you can get adequate quantities of these by taking a multivitamin tablet— something that is recommended for the Protein Express Diet, as well as the Atkins and Dukan diets. The real purpose of the green powder is to provide the other, less studied, substances that you obtain from eating vegetables like spinach, broccoli, peppers and kale. These chemicals, called phytochemicals are often associated with the vibrant colors of many fruits and vegetables. Phytochemicals have antioxidant properties, and are thought to be responsible for many of the health benefits of a diet that includes significant amounts of colorful vegetables and fruit. Increased consumption of green vegetables has consistently been shown to be associated with lower rates of chronic conditions such as heart disease and cancer.

Again, we can ask the whole foods vs. powders question. Am I suggesting that using a green supplement powder is as effective as eating fresh vegetables on a regular basis? No, of course not. For the Protein Express Diet I recommend that you eat fresh or frozen non-starchy, low calorie vegetables like spinach and broccoli as often as possible. (The Dukan diet is more restrictive and this is may be another good argument for using green powder).

The reality is that consuming green vegetables on a routine basis—especially at breakfast and lunch—is not easy, and most people simply don't do it. Green supplement powder contains the extract of a variety of beneficial plants, some of which you might not have occasion to eat at all. I think including this component dramatically increases the nutritional value of your meals, especially when time is limited or when you are eating on the run. There is no need to make the perfect the enemy of the the good: use green supplement powder in your drinks as a sort of nutritional safety net, and continue to consume fresh, non-starchy vegetables as often as you can. As with protein powders, I will make some specific suggestions for green powder in the next section.

The final, and optional, component for the Protein Express diet drinks is psyllium powder. Powder produced from psyllium seed husks is an easy and inexpensive way to consume more fiber. Fiber comes from the non-digestible portions of the plants that we eat and is important to digestion. People who eat a low carbohydrate / high protein diet are often subject to constipation without an added fiber source. Even many people who eat "normally" do not get sufficient fiber in advanced countries.

The best known brand of psyllium powder is Metamucil—which is sold as a fiber source and/or laxative. Any supermarket or drug store chain will also have less expensive store brands You can add a teaspoon or so of psyllium powder to your drinks on an as-needed basis depending on whether or not you experience constipation.

The Dukan diet instead recommends daily consumption of oat bran as a fiber source. Oat bran is a bit harder to find and does not work as well in drinks, but you can substitute this if you prefer it to psyllium powder. **NOTE**: YOU CAN EAT OAT BRAN DIRECTLY FROM THE BOX IF YOU WISH, BUT NEVER TRY THIS WITH PSYLLIUM POWDER: THIS CAN CAUSE CHOKING. ALWAYS MIX PSYLLIUM THOROUGHLY WITH WATER.

EASY MEAL PREPARATION

The drinks used in the Protein Express diet can be prepared in less than five minutes. I strongly recommend that you buy at least two packages of each component and keep one in your car or workplace. The primary advantage of this diet is that you always have a fast, easy and inexpensive alternative to diet-killing choices like fast food and vending machine snacks.

As noted previously, there are three components to your meals: (1) protein powder, (2) "green" powder, and optionally (3) psyllium fiber powder. Always mix your drinks only with water. Do not use juice or milk (even skim milk). Doing so will invalidate your high-protein/low carb diet by adding carbohydrates and calories.

Always mix your own drinks. There are a number liquid, premixed products available, some of which claim to be high protein products. These are invariably formulated primarily for profitability. They contain far less protein and far more carbohydrate than the drinks you will mix yourself. Most of these liquid products are roughly the equivalent of skim chocolate milk with a vitamin pill added and perhaps a bit of extra protein. They are typically sugar-laden and expensive—and they certainly do not contain the bene-fits of the plant phytochemicals in the green powders I recommend.

Note that you do not have to mix all three components into one drink. If you don't like the idea of combining the green powder with the protein powder, then by all means feel free to mix two separate drinks; just be sure to use only water for each. If fact, one strategy that can be useful is to mix the psyllium powder (and perhaps the green powder) into a drink and consume it twenty minutes or so before the protein drink. This will help you feel more satisfied. I'll include more tips on how to use psyllium to make you drinks more filling later in this section.

SELECTING PROTEIN POWDERS

When choosing a protein powder, look for the following:

- Minimum 23 grams of protein per serving.
- Maximum 140 calories per serving.
- Maximum 2 grams of fat per serving.
- Maximum 1 gram of saturated fat per serving.
- No Trans-fat
- Maximum 5 grams of carbohydrate per serving.
- Avoid aspartame. Sweeteners such as Stevia and Su-cralose are preferable.

As long as you follow the guidelines above, and choose a product available from a reputable source, any protein powder you select should be effective. Protein powders are available in a number of flavors, such as chocolate, vanilla and strawberry.

SPECIFIC PRODUCTS

Here are three specific brands that I use myself:

OPTIMUM NUTRITION GOLD STANDARD PROTEIN POWDER - DOUBLE RICH CHOCOLATE

24 grams of protein

120 calories

2 grams of fat, 1 gram of saturated fat, no trans fat

3 grams of carbohydrate

Cost: Online at Amazon.com, $52.99 for 74 servings (5 pounds) or $0.76 per serving

Note: This product was was tested by Consumer Reports (July, 2010) and found to be within safe limits.

TRADER JOE'S SOY PROTEIN POWDER - VANILLA FLAVOR

25 grams of protein

120 calories

1 gram of carbohydrate

1.5 gram of fat, no saturated or trans fat

Cost: At Trader Joe's $14.99 for 30 servings (2 pounds) or $0.50 per serving

Note: This product was not tested by Consumer Reports (July, 2010).

BODY FORTRESS WHEY PROTEIN POWDER - CHOCO-LATE

26 grams of protein

140 calories

4 grams of carbohydrate

2 grams of fat, 1 gram saturated fat, no trans fat

Cost: At Wal-Mart, $14.99 for 27 servings (2 pounds) or $0.56 per serving

<u>Note</u>: This product was not tested by Consumer Reports (July, 2010).

I like to make my drinks with roughly half whey and half soy. I find that mixing chocolate flavored whey and vanilla flavored soy produces a good combination. If you look at the carbohydrate and fat content of the three products above, you'll notice that the soy powder has significantly less of both. Therefore, if you choose to follow a diet which is highly restrictive of carbohydrates (such as the initial phases of Atkins or Dukan), you may want to rely more heavily on soy powder.

While the three products above are good examples and are among the lowest cost per serving I have found, there are dozens of other worthy products out there. Feel free to shop based on cost and convenience as long as you are buying from a reputable outlet. One thing to keep in mind is that the nutritional values (for example grams of protein or calories) can be slightly different for the same product in different flavors.

GREEN POWDERS

In general, I'm a big fan of Trader Joe's products because of their low prices and reputation for high quality. The green powder that I use regularly is:

TRADER JOE'S VERY GREEN DRINK MIX

Ingredients include: Extract of alfalfa leaf, barley grass, spinach, broccoli, wheat grass, green tea, spirulina, and many more.

Serving size: 1 tablespoon / day

Calories: 30

Carbohydrate: 6 grams

Protein: 1 gram

Fat: none.

Cost: At Trader Joes' $10.99 for 35 servings or $0.31 per serving.

If I consume more than one protein drink per day, then I usually like to mix half of the 1-tablespoon per day serving into each drink. One tablespoon is equal to three teaspoons, so to do this, you would mix about a teaspoon and a half into each drink, and each drink would get half of the nutritional values listed above.

There are dozens of other green powders available. Common brands include "Green Vibrance," "Green SuperFood," and "Greens First." You can find these online or at health food stores like Whole Foods. Nearly all brands will include basic green vegetable extract from spinach, broccoli, etc. Some use only organic plants. Some include many more exotic ingredients.

Trader's Joe's Very Green, at $10.99 for 30 servings, is by far the most affordable powder I have found. Most other brands are priced from $20 to $50 for a one month supply. Trader Joe's also has a more upscale alternative called "Super Green Drink Mix" which sells for about $20 and has more and organic ingredients. There is also a "Super Red Drink Mix" that contains extract from red and blue colored fruits and vegetables. I like to alternate between the Very Green powder and the Super Red Drink mix powder to get the benefits of both green vegetables and colorful fruits in my protein drinks.

PSYLLIUM HUSK POWDER

The most well-known brand is Metamucil, but nearly every grocery and drug store has its own cheaper brand. I have used the one sold at Target. Make sure you choose a sugar-free version. I typically add about one teaspoon of powder to drinks on an interim/as-needed basis to avoid constipation. If you are consuming a very high protein diet and little in the way of vegetables, you will probably want to include this in every drink.

TIPS TO MAKE YOUR DRINKS THICKER/MORE FILLING

The protein drinks I suggest will generally be of liquid consistency: something similar to chocolate milk. If you'd like to make your drinks thicker, more filling, or simply add some variety, try these tricks:

- Mix about a teaspoon of psyllium powder, perhaps with the green powder, with water and drink it about 20 minutes or half an hour before making the protein drink. After drinking the psyllium drink, immediate drink another 1-2 glasses of water. The psyllium will absorb the water in your stomach and help you feel more full.
- Mix a teaspoon or so of psyllium powder with water in a glass. Then let it sit for 10-15 minutes. It will thicken as the psyllium absorbs the water. Next mix in the protein and green powder and still vigorously for a thicker more "shake-like" drink.
- Try mixing the drinks in advance and freezing. When you're ready to eat, you can thaw slightly to an ice-cream-like consistency. Alternatively, you can freeze the drink in a paper cup along with a Popsicle stick. Tear away the paper cup and you have a protein Popsicle.

STARTING YOUR DIET

Now that you know how to prepare the protein drinks that form the backbone of the Protein Express diet, all you have to do is follow some very easy steps to begin your weight loss program. You can use the techniques in this book in two basic ways: (1) You can follow the simple Protein Express diet steps laid out below, or (2) You can use the ideas in this book while following virtually any other diet: Dukan, Atkins, South Beach, or any low-fat/low-calorie diet.

The next section covers the steps in the diet I have devised. Later, I'll show you how to use protein shakes as part of your weight loss strategy if you are following virtually any other diet. The Protein Express Diet is divided into two simple phases: Weight Loss and Maintenance.

THE WEIGHT LOSS PHASE: 5 EASY STEPS

To begin your weight loss program, simply follow the five easy steps below. Your objective should be to consistently lose from 1-4 pounds per week while maintaining a healthy diet that includes all the necessary nutrients. You may well lose more weight at the beginning of the program, but much of this is likely to be water.

STEP 1

Substitute at least one—and preferably two—meals for a protein drink consisting of from 2 to 3 servings of protein powder. By far the easiest meal to do this with is breakfast. Nearly everyone is in a hurry at breakfast time, and a great many people make the mistake of eating too many carbohydrates (cereal, bagel, etc.), and too little protein.

Very few people consume green vegetables at breakfast, so a drink that includes green powder may offer an important nutritional boost. A drink that includes two servings (about 50 grams) of protein along with half the day's portion of green powder and perhaps some psyllium will come in at under 300 calories. This is roughly the same as a bagel—without the cream cheese. So you are getting a highly nutritious meal with very high protein, very low fat and carbohydrate, as well as low calories.

For maximum effectiveness, you can also replace a second meal, typically lunch. This may be harder, as you may have a strong desire for solid food by this time. If so, feel free to combine a high-protein solid food (for example, chicken breast without the skin), with a dessert protein drink.

However, you must be very strict in situations where no high-protein solid food is available. If the only other alternative is carbohydrate and fat-laden fast food, then instead prepare a larger protein drink with more servings. Use the techniques I described with psyllium to make your drink more filling. One of the primary benefits of the Protein Express diet is that it removes the excuse for going the fast food route by always having the ingredients for a liquid meal readily available.

Follow each protein drink with at least one additional glass of water, and remember to drink lots of water throughout the day. Recall that when your digestive system breaks down protein, it will create waste products that need to be flushed out of your system. Drinking plenty of water ensures that this goes smoothly.

STEP 2

Vitamin Supplementation: I strongly recommend consuming a daily multivitamin. I prefer the formula used in "Centrum Silver." This is marketed to adults over age 50, but I think it is a good choice for everyone. You can buy the brand name version, or there are a number of cheaper store brands available that offer the same formula.

One reason I like "Centrum Silver" is that it contains no iron. Men in particular need to be cautious about consuming too much iron. If you are using the Trader Joe's soy protein product, it already contains significant amounts of iron, so you do not need more. Some researchers believe that excess iron consumption may be partly responsible for the difference in lifespan between men and women because menstruation removes excess iron from women's bodies. Some men regularly give blood in hopes of achieving the same result.

In addition to the multivitamin, I also usually take 1-2 fish oil capsules each day. Research has shown that many people who consume Western diets are deficient in the omega-3 oils that are found in fish. Omega-3 fatty acids are crucial for brain function. Fish oil tablets are available everywhere; I have found that the Target brand is usually a good low cost alternative. Be sure that the brand you select indicates it has been purified to remove mercury.

STEP 3

For your remaining meal(s), consume only low-carbohydrate, high protein dishes, together with non-starchy, colorful vegetables. Do not eat fruit; it is too high in sugar. If you feel strongly that you want the nutritional benefits of fruit during the weight loss phase, try the Trader Joe's Super Red Drink mix powder or a similar product. Drink plenty of water with your meal.

I have included a list of foods you can feel free to enjoy, as well as a list of those you must avoid in the next section. If you want specific ideas for preparing your meals, you can follow the guidelines and recipes for either the Dukan diet or the Atkins diet. In general, I strongly prefer the more protein-intensive Dukan diet. If you do decide to incorporate significant fats and oils in your diet, I would strongly suggest that you limit yourself as much as possible to the so-called "good fats" (monounsaturated fats) such as olive oil, canola oil and peanut oil. At all costs avoid excessive saturated fat and, especially, trans fat.

Feel free to follow up your meal with another protein drink. As I noted earlier, this can go a long way toward giving you the sense of a "sweet dessert." That will help you avoid carb-craving and make it easier to stick with your diet.

STEP 4

Exercise! I strongly recommend that you include some sort of exercise in your plan. Later in this book, I describe the benefits of walking for exercise, and also give you some ideas for a "high intensity" approach that will allow you burn more fat within a given amount of time. I have also included a brief section with information on weight lifting and other resistance exercises. The point of this is to avoid loss of muscle during the weight loss phase. As I noted earlier, consuming more protein is very helpful in limiting the loss of lean tissue, but only exercise can ensure you don't lose lots of muscle. Again, exercise is optional, but highly recommended.

STEP 5

Monitor and Record. I strongly recommend weighing yourself every day. This will help keep you motivated, and once you get to the maintenance phase, it will help ensure you don't let your weight rebound. Weighing yourself daily will also give you a sense of the normal variation you can expect. Your weight will fluctuate within a few pounds but should gravitate downward over time. Always weigh yourself at the same time of day: the best time is right after waking up. Empty your bladder and then weigh yourself. This is the easiest time to get a consistent result.

While you should weigh yourself daily, I suggest only recording your weight weekly. Try to be as consistent as possible: Record your weight right after waking up on the same day of the week. It's better if you choose a day with a regular schedule so you will have had about the same amount of sleep the night before. I would suggest recording your actual weight, as well as the low and high weights for the week (I usually can remember these numbers, but if not, feel free to make a daily note somewhere). This will give you both a number and a range—something that will be very useful in the maintenance phase.

Another very useful thing you can do is record your body fat percentage. The easiest way to do this on a regular basis is with a bioimpedance body fat analyzer. These work by sending a very weak electric current through your body and then measuring the electrical resistance. Lean tissue conducts electricity better than fat, so the device is able to do a calculation that estimates your body fat percentage. Some bathroom scales have these devices built-in, or you can buy a hand-held one. I use the Omcron HBF-306C, which costs about $30 and is generally highly rated for its ease of use and accuracy.

Keep in mind that bioimpedance body fat analyzers have some real limitations. It is critical that you take measurements at a consistent time of day. For me, right after waking up is really the only viable option. The body fat percentage shown will vary as much as 4-5% throughout the day, because the amount of water you are retaining will change. Do not focus too much on the number shown: it is probably not especially accurate. The point is to record the number at consistent times and look for a downward trend. The calculation depends on your weight, so you will have to adjust this periodically.

While recording your weight and perhaps your body fat percentage gives you a numeric sense of your progress, you may also find it helpful to visualize the amount (or volume) of fat you are losing. It can be great motivator to actually see (and hold) a fairly accurate representation of the body fat you are eliminating.

The easiest way to visualize your fat loss is to visit the supermarket. Lean meat (muscle) has a density of about 1.06 g/ml, while fat has a density of around 0.9 g/ml. In other words, a pound of fat occupies about 18% more space than a pound of lean meat. So to imagine a pound of fat, find a one-pound package of lean meat and then visualize something about 18% bigger. Or you can look for a cut of meat that has plenty of fat and take that as a pretty conservative estimate; one good choice is vacuum packed bacon. If you want to be more exact and have a tangible motivator on hand at all times, you can also purchase an unpleasant looking plastic fat replica.

SUMMARY

That's it! Just follow those five steps and you will begin to see significant results. You can allow yourself one "cheat meal" per week without doing too much damage, but I would continue to exercise some degree moderation—and in particular try to avoid consuming large amounts of sugar and other refined carbohydrates, even during cheat meals. The reality is that these foods are simply not food for you in any amount, and it is best to get away from the idea that eating them is some sort of "reward."

During the weight loss phase, you should generally be highly motivated, and if you keep to the program, the scale (and the body fat analyzer) should give you positive results that reinforce that motivation. However, if you find that you nonetheless occasionally blow a meal and eat things that you should not (very often this will happen in the context of a social situation, such as eating out with friend or co-workers), you can use the "one-for-one reaction" strategy that I describe later in the section on the maintenance phase of your diet. This will give you a tool for immediately and proactively responding to occasional lapses.

Once again, here are the five simple steps for the Protein Express Diet Weight Loss Phase:

1. Replace 1 or 2 meals with a high protein, high nutrition drink. Also use a protein drink meal replacement anytime you might be tempted to resort to fast food or other poor choices. Keep the ingredients readily available at home and in your car/office. Drink more water after every protein drink.
2. Take a multivitamin and 1-2 fish oil capsules per day. I suggest a vitamin that does not include iron.

3. For the remaining meals, eat a high protein dish, non-starchy, colorful vegetables, and follow up with a protein drink dessert if desired. Drink water with every meal and throughout the day.
4. Exercise! Walking and, ideally, some form weight lifting or other strength building routine is highly recommended.
5. Monitor and Record. Weigh yourself daily, and record weekly. Take care to weigh yourself at consistent times, preferably right after waking up.

RECOMMENDED AND DIS-ALLOWED FOODS - WEIGHT LOSS PHASE

RECOMMENDED PROTEIN DISHES

Lean Beef (avoid ground beef, unless it is very lean)

Lean Pork (Canadian bacon is okay—regular is not)

Chicken and other poultry without the skin

All Fish

All Shellfish

Tofu

Eggs but avoid butter, fat or oil.

And, of course, protein powder drinks

RECOMMENDED   NON-STARCHY/COLORFUL
VEGETABLES

Artichoke

Asparagus

Bell Peppers

Broccoli

Brussels Sprouts

Cabbage

Carrots - especially raw

Celery

Cucumber

Eggplant

Green Beans

Kale

Mushrooms

Onions

Spinach

Tomatoes

Zucchini

Any other non-starchy vegetable with a very low glycemic index

NON ALLOWED DURING THE WEIGHT LOSS PHASE

Bread of any type, including whole grain.

Rice

Breakfast cereal of any kind.

Potatoes of any kind

Pasta of any kind

Processed snacks or chips of any kind.

Fruit or fruit juice (Try the Trader Joe's Super Red Drink Mix instead)

Milk, except a small amount in coffee or tea.

Beer

Any beverage except water, coffee, tea or wine (in moderation)

Any sugary desserts: cake, pie, ice cream, etc.

OPTIONAL: ACCELERATE YOUR WEIGHT LOSS WITH A PROTEIN FAST

It you are especially adventurous and would like to try a much more extreme technique, you can add a protein fast to your weight loss strategy. Fasting—or completely forgoing food of any kind—has, of course, long been associated with religious practice. More recently, fasting has become a much more mainstream technique for people interested in weight loss, detoxification and general health.

The duration of a fast can vary from a single day to as long as weeks or even months. Experience has shown that human beings are actually much more resilient to prolonged periods without food than most of us would expect. In fact, some proponents of paleolithic-style diets advocate intermittent fasting because our prehistoric ancestors would have often faced periods of food scarcity: at a basic level, humans may be biologically designed to endure fasts.

One of the best personal accounts of an extended fast I have seen appeared in the March, 2012, issue of *Harper's Magazine*. In the article "Starving your way to vigor: the benefits of an empty stomach," Steve Hendricks describes a fast that lasted a full twenty days. Hendricks consumed no food of any type for the entire duration of the fast and lost over twenty pounds. The article also offers a good historical overview of fasting, including the story of a 453 pound man who, in 1965, fasted for an entire year—and lost over 270 pounds. Hendricks also presents anecdotal evidence that fasting may be effective in treating a number of diseases, including diabetes, epilepsy and even cancer. However, virtually no formal research has been done in this area. (The Harper's article is available online, but a subscription is required.)

A major drawback of a full-fledged fast like the one that Hendricks underwent is that you will, almost without question, lose a significant amount of muscle along with fat. As we saw in the initial chapter of this book, consuming protein can help minimize that loss of lean tissue. Therefore, if you want to try fasting, I would strongly suggest that you undertake a "protein fast" where you continue to consume a minimal amount of protein, rather than forgoing food entirely.

The easiest way to do this is simply to limit yourself to a daily maximum of two of the protein drinks I've described here. Consume nothing else except water and perhaps black coffee or tea. If each drink contains two servings of protein powder, you would be taking in about 100 grams of protein per day. I strongly recommend that you also include the green supplement powder and take the daily vitamin and fish oil supplement. This will give you significant daily protein intake as well as the benefit of plant phytochemicals—all for no more that 500-600 calories per day.

A protein fast is obviously not for everyone. Make no mistake: this is an extreme dieting technique, and you should consult your physician before trying it. Nonetheless, it can be a valuable way to lose weight more rapidly. If you decide to try a protein fast, I would suggest beginning with a one-day fast. As you gain more experience, you can optionally extend the duration or perhaps engage in intermittent short fasts on a regular basis.

KICKING THE FAST FOOD AND PROCESSED SNACK HABIT

One of the most important arguments for my use of protein drinks in the Protein Express Diet is that it removes the normal excuse for relying on fast food or processed snacks, chips and the like. Protein powder is affordable and you can keep the ingredients readily available so you can have a healthy meal almost anywhere—and within a few minutes.

Your immediate response to this may be that a protein drink is simply not going to be as satisfying as a burger and fries. To some extent, the truth of this is inescapable: Fast food and snacks are designed to taste good and to satisfy. They are designed to be addictive—and therefore profitable.

It is very important to understand that eating unhealthy foods that taste good is not about nutrition; it is really a form of entertainment. We do it because we enjoy it. That's fine, but you have to understand the price you are paying for that entertainment. Is the cost really worth it?

One technique I would suggest so that you can begin to access the value or "reward" you get from eating fast food and snacks is to time your activities. The next time you eat fast food, keep track of how much time you spend waiting in line and for the food to be prepared. Then time how long it takes you to eat. Doing that allows you to put a number on the experience. How long does the "satisfaction" really last? Are you getting a good return on your entertainment money—and, much more importantly—on the cost in terms of your health?

You probably wouldn't be inclined to pay full price to watch a movie that lasted only 15 minutes. By keeping track of the time you spend actually eating fast food and snacks you can get a better handle on the trade-off you are making. How long does it take you to eat a cookie or a cupcake? How long does the "tastes good" sensation last? Is it worth it?

While a protein drink is probably never going to offer the same level of immediate gratification as a massive fast food meal, you can use the techniques I described previously (such as including psyllium husk powder), to make the drinks more satisfying. You will also find that the protein content makes the drinks more filling that you might expect—and of course, you will feel much better about yourself afterwards.

A second way to help get fast food craving under control is to really understand exactly what you are eating. For that, I would highly recommend the book (and also documentary movie) Fast Food Nation, which gives a great overview of the industry and tells the story of exactly how the food finds its way from the ranch or farm all the way to your plastic tray. Here's a classic quote from the part of the book that discusses the numerous cases where people have become ill (or even died) from eating fast food:

> The medical literature on the causes of food poisoning is full of euphemisms and dry scientific terms: coliform levels, aerobic plate counts, sorbitol, MacConkey agar, and so on. Behind them lies a simple explanation for why eating a hamburger can make you seriously ill: There is shit in the meat. (p. 197)

Think about it!

THE MAINTENANCE PHASE

If you stick with the five simple steps I outlined in the "Weight Loss" section and focus on consistently losing 1-2 pounds per week, you should have little difficulty reaching your goal. The real problem that nearly everyone runs into is maintaining their weight loss and avoiding the dreaded yo-yo effect. Because I believe that everyone is different and that some degree of experimentation is important in finding the optimal diet that works for you, I have incorporated two options into the maintenance phase of the Protein Express Diet; you can choose the option that best meets your needs and your philosophy regarding nutrition and the role that food plays in your life. There is little point in choosing to follow a long-term maintenance diet that is fundamentally at odds which what you most enjoy about eating; to do so is to set yourself up for failure.

Before describing the two maintenance options, I want to first give you an important rule that you should use with either option: The one-for-one reaction. This will give you a straightforward way to limit the damage on those (inevitable) occasions when you cheat.

THE ONE-FOR-ONE REACTION RULE

The rule is very simple: If you cheat significantly at a particular meal—in other words, if you eat significant quantities of foods (in particular, refined carbohydrates) that are not on the approved list for your diet—then you must immediately react by substituting at least one additional "normal" meal with a high protein drink consisting of two servings (about 50 grams) of protein powder.

For example, suppose that you typically have a protein drink for breakfast but eat "normal" foods for your other meals. On a particular occasion, you dine out with your co-workers and eat/drink substantial quantities of things that you know you shouldn't. The next day you need to immediately react by substituting one of your normal meals (for example, lunch) with a protein drink containing two servings of protein powder (or around 250-300 calories, if you also include the green powder). If you really go wild, then go ahead and substitute two meals.

The idea here is to have an easy and straightforward tool for responding to the inevitable lapses that will certainly occur. Anyone who participates in normal social activity and shares meals with others is likely to fall off the wagon occasionally. The key is to make sure it is occasional. Do not let this rule become an excuse for chronic cheating! That will lead you toward failure and regain of the weight you have lost.

MAINTENANCE PHASE OPTION 1: CONTINUED LOW-CARB / "PALEOLITHIC" DIET

If you find that you have adjusted to the high protein/low carbohydrate weight loss phase diet and no longer feel substantial craving for carbohydrates, then there are good reasons to simply stick with this basic plan. This is the choice that I have made. For me, the argument made by those who advocate a "paleolithic" diet that is geared toward those foods that ancient hunter-gatherers would have eaten is quite compelling. Humans are little changed in terms of basic biology since prehistoric times, and therefore, we should be able to thrive on the food types that were available before the dawn of agriculture.

One obvious question is: How can I possibly advocate using protein powder (and green powder) in a diet that purports to somehow be "prehistoric?" In truth, very few (maybe none) of the foods we eat today were available in prehistoric times. Modern vegetables are nearly all domesticated species that were bred by people. Likewise, today's cattle—even if grass-fed—bear little resemblance to the animals hunted by our prehistoric ancestors. Those animals would have lived in the wild, scrambled for food and lived in constant fear of natural predators. As a result, they likely would have carried far less fat than today's farm animals. The point is that, you should do the best you can to deliver the optimal basic nutrients to your body. I don't see any conflict in using modern innovations like protein powder, because nearly all the foods we eat are, by definition, non-natural innovations created by people over time.

My personal maintenance diet continues to focus on high protein intake. There is significant research showing that large amounts of saturated animal fat is simply not good for you and leads to long term problems. I therefore try to strictly limit (but not eliminate) saturated fat. Again, I think there is a good basis for doing this even if you believe strongly in a hunter-gatherer style diet because the animals eaten by our forebears would likely have been much leaner than the domesticated ones we consume today.

If you choose to use this option and continue a high protein and low carbohydrate maintenance diet, then follow these basic rules:

- Continue to use a protein / green powder drink for one meal per day.

- Always use the protein drink at times when the only other alternative is fast food, vending machines or snack foods.
- For other meals, eat the same same foods allowed in the weight loss phase.
- You can now add fruit to your diet. However, I strongly recommend choosing less sugary, lower calorie fruits, in particular berries. For example, blueberries are a better choice than mango.
- Low fat dairy products such as yogurt or cottage cheese are fine in moderation.
- Any non-starchy vegetable is fine.
- When selecting oils for cooking, try to use extra virgin olive or canola.
- Nuts are fine in moderation, but keep in mind that many nuts (such as almonds) are very high in calories and it can be very difficult to eat "just a few." Do not kid yourself that you can regularly indulge in large quantities of nuts and not gain weight.
- Wine (preferably red) and the occasional lite beer can be consumed in moderation.
- Avoid fruit juice (eat the whole fruit instead), sugared drinks, and soda of any kind. If you absolutely must drink soda, choose diet—but understand that even diet soda has been associated with weight gain
- Avoid all refined carbohydrates: bread, pasta, cakes, pies, chips, sugary snack foods and the like.
- Always use the "one-for-one reaction" rule if you cheat—but keep it occasional!
- Read The Dukan Diet and/or The New Evolution Diet for more ideas and recipes.

MAINTENANCE PHASE OPTION 2: "SMART" CARB / HIGH PROTEIN DIET

For a great many people, a long-term diet that tries to entirely avoid carbohydrates like bread and pasta is simply not going to be realistic or sustainable. If you are someone who truly enjoys these foods and simply cannot imagine giving them up indefinitely, then the "paleolithic" approach is not for you.

Instead, I recommend you follow a "smart" carb approach in which you carefully select and control your carbohydrate intake. This approach is very similar to the strategy advocated by Dr. Arthur Agatston in his book, The South Beach Diet, and I would strongly suggest reading this book for a great many good ideas and recipes for preparing foods that incorporate only healthy carbohydrates and fats.

The really key points for this diet are to confine yourself exclusively to whole grain breads and pasta, and to strongly emphasize the use of healthy fats and oils, such as olive, canola and peanut oil. It is critical that when you purchase bread or pasta products, you look specifically for the words "whole wheat" or "whole grain" on the package. Whole grain products are prepared using the entire seed—including the husk and other non-digestible components. This results in foods that have more fiber, digest more slowly and have a lower glycemic index.

Recall that the glycemic index is a measure of the speed with which carbohydrates result in increased sugar in your blood. In general, sugary and refined foods have a higher glycemic index than whole grains or non-starchy vegetables. White flour, which has been refined by removing all the parts of the wheat seed that are non-digestible, results in foods with extremely high glycemic indexes—for example, white bread actually causes your blood sugar level to increase faster than directly eating table sugar. You can find the glycemic index for any common food here: http://www.glycemicindex.com/.

 In general, you want to choose carbohydrates with a low or medium glycemic index—as long as you are making healthy, common sense choices rather than relying solely on the index. As we saw earlier, a candy bar that happens to have a moderate glycemic index does not count as a healthy choice. One important rule of thumb is to simply avoid any white-colored foods, including white bread, white rice and potatoes.

It's very important to realize that just because you eat only whole grain bread and pasta it does not mean you can eat excessive quantities. Eat in moderation, and stop when you are still slightly hungry. In general, you still want to make sure that your meals are relatively high in protein. Your meals should include foods like lean cuts of beef and pork, fish, eggs and tofu. Including more protein will help you fill more full and thus avoid overeating when it comes to bread and pasta. As always, you must avoid refined/processed carbohydrates, snack foods and sugary desserts. Instead, follow up your meal with a protein drink.

If you choose to use this option and go with a smart carb / high protein maintenance diet, then follow these basic rules:

- Continue to use a protein / green powder drink for one meal per day.
- Always use the protein drink at times when the only other alternative is fast food, vending machines or snack foods.

- For other meals, eat the same foods allowed in the weight loss phase.
- You can now add whole grain breads and pasta to your diet in moderation. Always view foods of this type as the "most dangerous" element of your regular meals.
- Low fat dairy products such as yogurt or cottage cheese are fine in moderation.
- You can now add fruit to your diet. However, I strongly recommend choosing less sugary, lower calorie fruits, in particular berries. For example, blueberries are a better choice than mango.
- Any vegetable is fine, except white potatoes. If you eat yams or sweet potatoes, use moderation.
- When selecting oils for cooking, try to use extra virgin olive or canola.
- Nuts, are fine in moderation, but keep in mind that many nuts (such as almonds) are very high in calories and it can be very difficult to eat "just a few." Do not kid yourself that you can regularly indulge in large quantities of nuts and not gain weight.
- Wine (preferably red) and the occasional lite beer can be consumed in moderation.
- Avoid fruit juice (eat the whole fruit instead), sugared drinks, and soda of any kind. If you absolutely must drink soda, choose diet—but understand that even diet soda has been associated with weight gain.
- Avoid all refined carbohydrates: white bread, cakes, pies, sugary snack foods and the like.
- Always use the "one-for-one reaction" rule if you cheat— but keep it occasional!
- Read The South Beach Diet for more ideas and recipes.

The two strategies above are broad enough to work with nearly any mainstream diet. Even if you choose to move to a more traditional low-fat diet plan, virtually any credible expert is likely to agree that you should avoid refined carbohydrates and instead focus on whole grains, lean proteins and healthy fats. You should feel free to pick the approach that works best for you, or formulate your own hybrid approach. For example, you might decide to limit whole grain bread and pasta to one meal per day (or a few days per week) and otherwise follow a low carb approach. The key is to find what works best for you.

THE YO-YO AVOIDANCE STRATEGY: DRAWING A LINE IN THE SAND

In the previous section, I gave you two basic strategies for a long term maintenance diet. The reality is that everyone is different, and you will need to experiment to find the permanent lifestyle diet that will allow you maintain your weight. It is critical to remember that preventing weight gain is only one important goal: you also have to enjoy your life! If you select a maintenance diet that is too rigid or restrictive, it's likely you'll eventually decide that the trade-off simply isn't worth it.

Specific people have different metabolisms and a unique sensitivity to carbohydrates. The only way you will find the right long-term strategy for you is to experiment. This is true even if you follow a very popular diet that has been scientifically evaluated using hundreds of people. Such studies result in average conclusions. While most people may have success on a given diet, there will always be some individuals who do not do well with a particular approach. How can you know in advance that you won't be one of those unlucky people? The only way to find out for sure is with some degree of trial and error.

The problem is that having invested the time, effort and willpower to lose your weight, you will understandably be very hesitant to take any chances that might result in regaining those pounds. But being too cautious can leave you vulnerable to complete abandonment of your diet as time passes and your enthusiasm wanes. It's much better to find the strategy that really works for you so your diet can truly become a lifestyle choice rather than an enduring restriction.

In order to feel free to experiment and try different maintenance approaches, it is vital that you have specific techniques you know you can rely on to quickly reverse any weight gain. This will give you the confidence you need to find the best long term approach for you.

 The first tool you can use to avoid regain weight has been covered already: the one-for-one reaction. If you blow a meal—and in particular if you eat the really forbidden things like sugary/processed/refined snacks, white bread, etc.—then you should immediately respond by replacing at least one regular meal with a protein drink containing two servings of protein (max 300 calories). If you really go to excess, replace two meals.

Beyond that, I will outline a very specific technique you can use to monitor your weight and respond immediately if you begin to gain. The importance of this cannot be overemphasized. There is nothing more demoralizing that gaining back most or all of the weight you have lost and then having to face starting again from scratch. And this can happen to anyone!

The key is to draw a line in the sand and respond immediately to any significant weight gain. That way, you only have to lose a few pounds, and you can do it quickly and with confidence. Don't put yourself in the position of having to work for weeks just to get back to where you started!

HOW TO DRAW A LINE IN THE SAND

As I mentioned earlier, you should make a habit of weighing yourself every day and recording your weight weekly. You should also record the high and low for the week. You can use those records to calculate an "action threshold" for you weight. If you reach that threshold you must, immediately take action to drive your weight back down where it belongs.

Here's how to calculate your "action threshold" or line in the sand:

1. Over a two week period during which your weight is relatively stable , take the five highest daily values for your weight. Make absolutely certain that you are weighing

ourself at consistent times of the day—preferably first thing in the morning.
2. Average those five high values (add them up and divide by 5).
3. Add a reasonable buffer to that average value. I would suggest 1-2 pounds. Remember, that the greater the buffer you choose, the more work you will have to do to get back to your target weight.
4. This is now your line in the sand. If, on any day, you weigh yourself and your weight hits or exceeds this weight, you must take immediate action!

WHAT TO DO IF YOU HIT YOUR LINE IN THE SAND:

1. Replace two meals with a protein drink consisting of 2 servings of protein for at least two days, preferably three or more. For your remaining meal, eat only protein-rich, low carbohydrate whole foods as recommended in the weight-loss phase of the diet.
2. Immediately return to the weight-loss phase and stay there until your weight drops consistently below the average high that you calculated. Note: your weight must consistently be below the average that you calculated—not the average plus the buffer.
3. You can then return to a maintenance strategy.

When you return to the maintenance phase, it is critical to evaluate things. Was your weight gain due to simply blowing your diet and eating the wrong foods? If so, you can probably return to more or less the same strategy and be more careful in the future. If your problem was eating sugary snacks, be sure to substitute protein drinks when you want something sweet.

If on the other hand, you were faithful to your diet but gained weight anyway, then you will need to modify your strategy. If you were eating significant quantities of whole grain carbs, then you may well be sensitive to these foods: you will have to push your diet more in the low carb direction. Try limiting foods like whole grain bread and pasta to one meal per day, or a couple of days per week. Monitor your weight carefully and be ready to take action again if you hit your line in the sand.

USING THE PROTEIN EXPRESS DIET TOGETHER WITH DUKAN, ATKINS OR ALMOST ANY OTHER DIET

The protein drinks used in the Protein Express diet have the advantage of being high in protein, low in both carbohydrates and fat, and also low in calories. This means that they will fit perfectly into virtually any diet — regardless of the particular philosophy or approach. Perhaps the most important benefit of using these protein drinks is speed and convenience. Regardless of how you feel about the use of protein powder in general, you will probably agree that these drinks are a better choice that most fast food or snacks you might find in a convenience store or vending machine. This is especially true if you include the green power, which offers the benefit of nutrients that are definitely not going to be found in other options. Therefore, you should keep the ingredients for these drinks handy for times when you have no other alternative.

A second important advantage is that these drinks will help skew your diet toward more protein intake. As we saw earlier, research suggests that consuming more protein while in the process of losing weight will help you avoid loss of muscle and other lean tissue. Exercise is, of course, also highly recommended to help maintain muscle mass.

If you are one a very strict diet, you can customize your protein drinks slightly if necessary. For example:

- If you are following a diet that is very restrictive of carbohydrates, such as the "induction phase" of the Atkins diet or phase one of the Dukan diet, you may want to skew your protein drinks toward soy rather than whey, because this typically contains less carbohydrate.
- The green powder also adds a small amount of carbohydrate. I strongly recommend that the green powder be included over the long term, but you can skip it for relatively short periods or on specific days (for example, phase two of the Dukan diet allows vegetables only every other day).

RULES FOR USING PROTEIN EXPRESS DRINKS WITH ANY OTHER DIET:

- I recommend continuing to use a protein / green powder drink for one meal per day.
- Always use the protein drink at times when the only other alternative is fast food, vending machines or snack foods.
- Always use the "one-for-one reaction" rule if you cheat— but keep it occasional!
- Follow the plan in the "Yo-Yo Avoidance Strategy" section once you get into the maintenance phase of your preferred diet. Draw your line in the sand and hold to it!
- Otherwise, follow the rules for your preferred diet.

A VEGAN/VEGETARIAN VERSION OF THE PROTEIN EXPRESS DIET

One of the advantages of the protein powder-based approach is that the Protein Express Diet can be used within a vegan or vegetarian framework. This contrasts with the Dukan Diet, for example, which is really not viable for non meat eaters.

If your vegetarian diet allows dairy products, then you can create your protein drinks using both whey and soy, since whey is a dairy product. For strict vegans, soy protein is the only option. Since you will necessarily be consuming a lot of soy protein powder on this diet, be absolutely certain to purchase a quality product from a reputable source. You may prefer to buy two different soy products from different sources and mix the two together as a way to enhance safety.

RULES FOR USING PROTEIN EXPRESS DRINKS WITH VEGAN OR VEGETARIAN DIETS:

- I recommend continuing to use a protein / green powder drink for at least one meal per day.
- Add protein drinks to your other meals as necessary to ensure you are getting substantial amounts of protein. This is especially important for vegans.
- I strongly recommend eliminating starchy vegetables during the weight loss phase of your diet. Emphasize non-starchy vegetables and tofu. Limit grains as much as possible—including even whole grain foods.
- Avoid any sugary fruit. Fruits with low glycemic indexes, such as apples, can be eaten in moderation during the weight loss phase.
- Follow the plan in the "Yo-Yo Avoidance Strategy" section once you get into the maintenance phase of your preferred diet. Draw your line in the sand and hold to it!

CONCLUSION

If you follow the two phases I have outlined for the Protein Express Diet, you should be able to make consistent progress toward your weight loss goal, and then successfully keep the weight off. Alternatively, you can follow the guidelines for nearly any other reasonable diet—although I recommend a low-carb approach, and particularly the Dukan Diet—and incorporate the protein drinks I have described as way to make food preparation easier and more flexible.

Some people may question my reliance on the use of protein drinks. I want to emphasize that I am in no way advocating a full-liquid diet; I recommend that a maximum of two meals per day be replaced with protein drinks. If you have the time and energy to prepare protein-rich whole food meals with fresh non-starchy vegetables, then by all means do it!

However, for most of us, when the boss is breathing down our necks, or when the kids need to be picked up, or when a myriad of other time pressures come into play, it may simply be impossible to prepare more than one healthy, protein-rich whole food meal per day. When time and access to healthy foods is limited, I feel strongly that the protein drinks I have described offer an optimal solution. If you follow the guidelines I have laid out—mix two types of protein, and incorporate green supplement powder and possibly fiber into your drinks—you will end up with meals that are nutritionally far superior to either whole foods that can be obtained quickly while you are on the run or commercial premixed liquid diet products.

The remainder of this book includes some additional information that will help you "turbo charge" your diet and potentially incorporate the ideas in this book into a long-term program for optimal health. The next chapter includes a very concise overview of the two most important types of exercise you can make a part of your lifestyle: walking and some form or weight lifting or resistance exercise. Finally, I have included a brief look at thermal dieting techniques.

CHAPTER 3: EXERCISE: EASY TIPS AND TECHNIQUES

EXERCISE, DIET AND THE TRUTH ABOUT WEIGHT LOSS

While the Protein Express Diet will certainly be effective by itself, I strongly recommend that you incorporate exercise into both your weight loss plan and your extended lifestyle. Exercise is a highly effective way to turbocharge your diet so that you lose more fat in a shorter period of time. If you choose to follow a simple and easy weight lifting program, you will also be doing everything possible to insure that you lose only fat—and not muscle or other critical lean tissue.

While exercise is a great way to add effectiveness to your diet strategy, it is important to realize right from the start that exercise by itself will likely NOT get the job done—at least not with the kind of measurable progress that will keep you motivated. Losing significant weight via exercise alone is a challenge because most of the foods we eat are very energy-intensive, and our bodies are very efficient at getting a lot of work from that energy intake.

For example, unless you weigh over 200 pounds, walking a mile will probably expend significantly less than 100 calories. That's not even equivalent to one 12-oz soda or light beer. A pound of fat equates to about 3500 calories, so you would probably need to walk well in excess of 35 miles (perhaps as far as 50 miles) just to burn off one pound. A trained marathon runner—who is by definition very efficient in his or her energy expenditure—probably only burns about 100 calories per mile or a total of 2600 calories over the 26-mile course. That's not even enough to lose a pound of fat!

The point is that exercise is a great way to maximize fat loss, minimize lean tissue loss, and—most importantly—improve your cardiovascular and general health. It is not however, by itself, a way for most people to quickly lose significant amounts of fat. Modifying your diet is by far the most important thing you must do to lose weight.

WALKING FOR FITNESS AND PLEASURE

Walking is, in the opinion of most experts, far and away the best fat-burning exercise for most people to incorporate into their lifestyle. Walking is arguably the most natural of all physical exercises for human beings, and it is accessible to nearly everyone. Even people who have extreme weight problems and low levels of general fitness can begin with a graduate walking program.

Walking exercises nearly all of the largest muscles in your body, including the the gluteal (butt) muscles, the quadriceps (the large, front muscles in your thigh), the hamstrings (the muscles in the back of your thigh), the hip flexors and the calf muscles. Walking can also bring the abdominal muscles and even the arm and shoulder muscles into play to some extent. Walking at a brisk pace also exercises the most important muscle in your body—your heart—and walking regularly will enhance your cardiovascular health significantly, compared with a sedentary lifestyle.

If you walk at a relatively brisk pace (at least 3.5 to 4 miles per hour) you will probably expend from 60-100 calories per mile. The exact number will depend primarily on your weight. You can easily find tables on the Internet that purport to give you an exact figures for calorie expenditure based on your weight and speed. However, I would advise against relying too heavily on such exact numbers. The reality is that the amount of energy you burn walking will probably depend on a number of factors and may vary significantly. The best strategy is simply to set a consistent goal—such as walking an average of half an hour or an hour a day, or several times per week—and then stick with it.

Remember that the primary goal for your walking program should be to improve and maintain your general health. Any extra weight loss is an added benefit. Medical research has consistently shown that people who engage in regular walking enjoy better health and are less prone to diabetes, heart disease and other chronic conditions.

While there are obviously many types of exercise you can engage in, for most people, a regular walking program has substantial advantages. For example:

- Studies have shown that walking briskly conveys most of the cardiovascular benefits of much more intense exercises, such as jogging. If you are someone who truly enjoys jogging or running, then by all means do it. However, if like me, you find it to be a thoroughly unenjoyable grind, then there is really no good reason to jog rather than walk. By choosing an activity that you enjoy, you will dramatically increase the likelihood that you will stick with the program.

- Walking is much lower impact and easier on the joints than running or many other active exercises. The probability of injury is much lower.

- When you walk it is easy to simultaneously engage in other activities—such as listening to music or an audio book. This makes your exercise program more time-effective because you can do two things you enjoy at once.

- You can walk almost anywhere and incorporate it into your lifestyle in very flexible ways. For example, a decision to leave the car at home, or even to consistently park at the outer-edge of the lot and then walk to your destination can have a significant cumulative effect over time.

- Walking requires no investment in special equipment; nor do you need to change into gym clothes. Just do it!

- Walking is by far the easiest exercise to enjoy with friends and family, because nearly everyone can do it.

TIPS TO GET THE MOST OUT OF YOUR WALKING PROGRAM

VARY YOUR ROUTE AND ROUTINE

It's a good idea to set an overall goal for the amount of time or distance you'll spend walking; for example, you might try to average half an hour or an hour per day, depending on the amount of time you have available. However, you don't need to hold the same daily routine. Try skipping a day and then walking twice as far the next day. You can lay out different routes of different distances near your home in order to inject constant variety into your walking (see below). This will help keep things interesting. Varying your exercise plan may even be more effective in terms of the health benefits you get: In The New Evolution Diet Arthur De Vany argues that exercise should he highly variable rather than routine and consistent because this does a better of job of replicating the natural lifestyle of our prehistoric ancestors.

USE GOOGLE MAPS TO DESIGN YOUR WALKING ROUTES

Google Maps offers a great tool for laying out alternate walking routes near your home, or in other locations when you travel. To measure the distance of a particular walking route follow these steps:

1. Navigate to http://maps.google.com and enter your home address to get a local map.
2. Now you need to turn on the distance measuring feature. I in the left pane, look toward the bottom and click the "Maps Labs" link just above the copyright notice. The Maps Labs screen will appear.
3. Click the option to enable the Distance Measurement Tool at the top. Then click Save Changes.
4. At the bottom left corner of the map, click the "ruler" icon. The left column will now display measurement options. You may want to select English, rather than metric
5. Click the starting point for your walking route. A green balloon will appear at that location.
6. Click subsequent points on the route—generally you'll want to click at every location where you need to make a turn.
7. Each time you click a new point, the total distance will show up in the left pane. You can use the Delete and Re-

set buttons on the left to remove the last point or start over at any time.

"READ" A BOOK WHILE YOU WALK

One of the great things about walking is that you can easily engage in other activities while you walk. If you enjoy music, you can, of course, carry a portable MP3 player or iPod. Another great option is to listen to an audio book. Like many busy people I often struggle to find the time to read, and I've found that combining reading and waking is a very efficient use of time.

The advent of downloadable audio books has made listing to a book much easier and more affordable that in the days when audio books were available only on CD. If you're interested in making a habit of "reading" while walking, I'd strongly recommend joining Audible.com.

Audible, which is a subsidiary of Amazon, currently offers membership programs that give you one audio book per month for $14.95. You generally also get one or two free books when you first sign up. This is a good deal if you'll listen to at least one book per month, since most books are priced higher than this. Audible generally has bestsellers as soon as they are released in printed form.

At the time of this writing, Audible.com was offering

special discounts for new members.

You may find that making a commitment to listen to books while walking and then joining a monthly book membership actually helps you keep with your walking program, since you'll be paying for that one book per month. To get the most for your money, try to select longer books; this will give you more hours of listening for the same price and will also make it easier to stick with a long book that might be harder to finish in printed form.

Another alternative for downloadable audio books is your local library. Many libraries now offer ebooks (both audio and text format). One of the most common services is Overdrive, which provides ebook capability to a large number of local and school libraries. If your library offers downloadable audio books, you should be able to access them from the library website. (You can search for a nearby library that offers the Overdrive service here: http://search.overdrive.com/.)

HIGH INTENSITY WALKING—A NEW STRATEGY

Over the course of many years of walking for exercise, I've developed my own strategy for increasing the intensity of my program, in order to burn more fat and build more muscle. The idea first occurred to me when my walking route took me past a new car dealership. I stopped to browse and began to focus on the miles per gallon numbers included on the window stickers.

Everyone knows, of course, that nearly all cars get better mileage on the highway than in the city. But why is this? To some extent it seems counter-intuitive. Travelling at a higher speed must certainly use more energy than travelling at a lower speed. This was, after all, one of the rationales for the 55 mile per hour speed limit that was enacted in the 1970s during the oil crisis.

The fact that higher speeds require more energy is especially evident if you consider the role of air resistance. As a car's speed increases, the air resistance it faces increases not in proportion to the speed, but as the cube of the speed. In other words, if you triple your speed—say from 20 mph to 60 mph—the air resistance holding back the car will increase not by 3 times, but by 3 X 3 X 3 or 27 times. And yet, even given this reality, cars still get better mileage on the highway.

So why is city mileage so poor? It's because of all the stop and go driving—and in particular because of the constant need for acceleration. Studies have shown that as much as 60% of the fuel you burn in city driving is used during acceleration; this is the hardest work that the engine does because it has to move the entire mass of the car from a dead stop and get it moving. On the highway, the car's momentum helps to propel it forward so that the car needs less energy per mile, even in the face of dramatically higher air resistance.

To use more energy, and therefore burn more fat, while walking, you can try to replicate city, as opposed to highway, driving. In other words, you need to vary your rate and focus especially on acceleration. This takes momentum out of the equation and forces your muscles to expend energy getting your body mass moving.

85

Here's the basic technique that I use to add intensity to my walking. I don't do this continuously, but rather use it for just a portion of the route:

1. Starting with a normal brisk walking space, slow to a much lower speed. Do not stop completely, but slow enough so that your forward momentum is dramatically reduced. Slow in a controlled fashion using your muscles, rather than putting pressure on your joints. Let your muscles expend energy to slow you down gradually; this will burn more fat and reduce the risk of injury.

2. Maintain that much slower pace for a few seconds—long enough to ensure that your momentum has been broken.

3. Now go immediately into full acceleration mode. Think in terms of a car doing a "jackrabbit" start from stop sign. The key is to get back to a brisk walk as rapidly as possible. This acceleration phase will burn fat and also help maintain or build muscle mass. If you've seen photos of Olympic sprinters, you know that these athletes generally have highly developed leg and lower body muscles—much more so than distance runners, who tend to have a scrawny appearance. Those sprinter's muscles are built by acceleration. You're trying to replicate that, although obviously in a less intense way.

4. Maintain the brisk pace for at least 60 seconds or so—then repeat.

Repeating this procedure—and consciously focusing on the acceleration phase—will add a lot of intensity to your exercise. You can gradually add this to your normal walking routine; try the technique during one leg of your route, and then increase the percentage of time you spend in "high intensity" mode over time. Don't maintain the slow pace for more than a few seconds because doing so will reduce the cardiovascular benefit of your walk—instead drive directly back into the acceleration phase. When you get tired, simply switch back to a continuous brisk walk.

Use this technique to add intensity to your walks, but don't feel you need to overdo it. Adding more intense exercise two or three times a week for a portion of you walk may be sufficient. Don't take things so far that your walking experience becomes unenjoyable—remember that the most important point is to incorporate regular exercise into your lifestyle.

QUICK AND EASY WEIGHT TRAINING

In this section I will offer a very basic overview of weight training exercises for people who are primarily interested in maintaining muscle mass and general fitness. My assumption is that you are NOT someone who truly enjoys lifting weights and wants to spend large amounts of time in the gym. Instead, I'll offer some basic tips for getting the most out of the minimum investment of time and energy. There are two basic questions that I'll try to answer here: (1) How should you structure your workouts in terms of repetitions and sets? and (2) What specific exercises should you do?

HOW MANY SETS SHOULD YOU DO?

Weight lifting exercise is generally divided into repetitions (or reps) and sets. So you might lift a weight ten times (ten reps). Then you will rest briefly and begin again. Each group of repetitions is called a set.

One of the biggest debates in weight lifting circles concerns the number sets that need to be performed. One group advocates a "one set to failure" strategy, while others advocate performing as many as five or even ten sets of the same exercise. A number of formal research studies have been done to try find out which approach works best for most people. Typically these studies have two groups of people perform either a one-set or a multi-set routine and then measure and compare strength gains for the two groups.

While a number of studies have been done, there is still no real consensus on the answer. Part of the problem is that the studies vary widely in terms of the people employed and in particular whether or not they had previous weight training experience. This is important because it is well known that people who begin lifting weights for the first time typically show fairly rapid strength improvement. It is not unusual for beginners to increase their strength by 50% or more within a short time. Much of this initial improvement is due to increased efficiency in the nervous system rather than a change in muscle mass; the first response to weight training is that your body simply gets better at mobilizing the muscle you already have.

Most studies that I have seen indicate that for people without significant prior weight training experience, one set is often just as effective as multiple sets. Obviously, if you are not someone who craves the gym, this is good news since you may be able to get away with less lifting. However, there is also evidence to suggest that after six months or so, a single set approach may be likely to result in a plateau for many people, especially if you are not able to maintain a very high level of intensity for that single set.

One of the better research studies I have seen was performed at the University of Hawaii and published in 2001. It focused on women with basic prior weight training experience who were divided into single-set and three-set groups. The women performed exercises under supervision over a six week period and the results were measured. The study found that for most exercises, the three-set approach resulted in significantly more strength gains. To find the study online, google "Single Multiple-Set Strength Training in Women hawaii.edu".

In the study above, both groups of women performed the exercises "to failure." This means that you continue performing repetitions to the point of failure, and it is very important that this be done with serious intensity. Especially if you are using the one-set approach, you must keep exercising until you reach the point where you absolutely, physically cannot advance the weight. At the point of failure you should hold the weight in place for several seconds—in other words, you should keep pushing (or pulling) even after it becomes evident you will not be able to complete the repetition. It is probably this last failed repetition that really drives the progress you will make.

When you perform intense weight bearing exercise, it will actually cause microscopic damage to your muscle fibers. If you then rest adequately between exercise sessions, your body will repair that damage and also make your muscles stronger in the process. This is the reason that it is critical to take at least 1 to 2 days rest between weight training exercises that employ the same muscle groups. It is, of course, also critical to have sufficient protein intake, so your blood supply will have adequate amino acid building blocks to support the muscle repair and strengthening process.

A second question is how many repetitions you should perform for each set. The general approach is to try to add one or more repetitions for each exercise until you reach a maximum. At that point you should add more weight. In the study above, the women performed 6-9 repetitions; in other words, once they were able to lift the weight 9 times, they added more weight in the next session. My personal preference is to advance the weight when I reach 10 repetitions. 12 is also a commonly used maximum.

In general, for any weight training exercise you should try to keep the repetitions per set roughly in the 5-12 range. This range has been shown to produce optimal gains in strength and muscle mass/tone. If you choose lighter weights and perform more than 12-15 reps you are getting into the range where the emphasis will be on endurance rather than strength or muscle gain.

The exact numbers you choose may have to be adapted to the equipment you are using. Many weight machines only allow you to add weight in 10 pound increments. So, for example, suppose you decide to try to keep your reps in the 6-9 range. If you are able to perform 9 repetitions with a weight of 50 pounds, then you would add 10 pounds at your next session. This is fine as long as you are then able to complete at least 5 reps with the new heavier weight. However, if you find you can only perform 3 or 4 reps, then it is probably better to reduce the weight and use a higher maximum (for example 12), so that you can keep the reps in the optimal range. In some cases you may find that you need to use a different repetition range for different exercises.

MY RECOMMENDATIONS

So putting all this information together, here are my specific recommendations:

- In general, three sets to failure is probably better than one set, especially once you have some experience and if you want to maximize the strength and muscle gains you get from your exercise. (Read the study I referenced above for specific some ideas.)
- If you are just beginning, or if you have no desire to add muscle and only want to prevent muscle loss while you are dieting, then a one-set routine should be effective for you. You can always change to a multi-set routine if you plateau at some point in the future.
- DO NOT lift weights to failure the first time you go into a gym. Take it easy and experiment to find the proper

weight that will get you in the 5-12 reps range. Don't over do it the first time. You will very likely be quite sore afterwards. If so, feel free to take several days or a week to recover before lifting again.

- Always repeat until failure and try to be as intense as possible about it. This where your progress will come from.
- If you do multiple sets, rest for 2 minutes between sets. Rest for 2-3 minutes between different exercises.
- Always take at least one day off between weight lifting sessions. I recommend at least two days of rest between exercising the same muscles. As you progress and get stronger, it may be necessary to rest for longer periods. Remember that you build muscle between sessions while you are resting The protein drinks you consume on the Protein Express diet will be help support this process.
- There is no appreciable difference between lifting weights to get strong/build muscle mass and weight training to get "toned." Women do not have the testosterone necessary for large muscles and, except in very rare cases, do not need to worry about becoming "muscle bound." Even most men probably do not have the genetics for really large muscle development. Lifting lighter weights for more receptions will increase endurance, but it will not be as effective in giving your muscles a toned appearance. So stay with the heaviest weights you can manage in the 5-12 repetition range.

WHAT EXERCISES SHOULD YOU DO?

The exercises you choose will depend on the equipment you have available. Obviously, if you have access to a commercial gym, you will have a lot more options. However, I have tried to emphasize exercises that can be performed on the more modest equipment often available at fitness centers in workplaces or apartment/condo complexes.

I strongly suggest using weight machines rather than free weights if possible. While serious bodybuilders and weightlifters may prefer dumbbells and barbells, for the rest of us machines are much safer and easier to work with. One especially important advantage of machines is that they allow you to work out alone—without a safety partner or "spotter."

As we saw in the previous section, a program that results in significant fat loss and muscle building (or at least preservation) really requires that you use relatively heavy weights. This means that purchasing free weights to use at home would be expensive, and exercising without a safety partner would be dangerous. If you do not have access to weight machines either at work or at home, I would strongly recommend investing in a gym membership if possible.

The exercises listed below are the ones I recommend for the best overall fitness and strength building program. All of these exercise are "compound." In other words, they use multiple joints and exercise major muscle groups, rather than focusing on a single muscle (for example your biceps). Compound exercises should always constitute the core of your training program, even if at some point you also choose to add single muscle (or "isolation") exercises.

I have not included instructions for the exercises here. There is little point to that since high quality instructional videos are available for virtually all exercises on YouTube. These are generally produced by professional trainers. I would suggest watching at least two different videos by different instructors for each exercise; this will give you a good sense of how to properly perform the exercise. If, as I recommend, you are using machines, then when you search for videos on YouTube, you may want to specify that to avoid seeing free weight exercises. For example, search for "machine bench press" rather than just "bench press." Obviously, if you are a member of a commercial gym then you should also seek out assistance from the trainers available onsite.

RECOMMENDED WEIGHT TRAINING EXERCISES

Bench Press: This will develop the major muscles in your chest (pectorals) as well as the triceps muscles in your arms. I suggest performing this exercise at a slight incline rather than completely flat for increased safety. Never perform this alone if you are using free weights rather than a machine.

Shoulder (or Military) Press: This will develop the major muscles in your shoulders (deltoids) as well as your triceps and upper back. Never perform this alone if you are using free weights rather than a machine.

Lat Pull Down: This will develop the major muscles in your upper back as well as the biceps muscles in your arm. You can use either a overhand or underhand grip. An underhand grip brings your biceps more into play.

Leg Press: The leg press machine will exercise all the major muscles in your upper legs, as well as your glutes (butt). Leg press machines are usually only available in larger gyms. If you don't have access to a leg press machine, you can substitute **leg extensions** and **leg curls**. These are isolation rather than compound exercises, but the machines are much more likely to be found in smaller gyms and fitness centers.

Those four or five exercises should be sufficient to give you a good whole body workout and help preserve and build your major muscle groups. There are, of course, dozens of other exercises, but if you are just getting started, I suggest focusing on the most important ones. As you progress, you can optionally add additional exercises, including isolation movements for your arms, abdominals, etc. Take things gradually and focus on putting together a training routine that you can stick with. It much better to stay with a program consisting of only a few major exercises than to end up abandoning something more ambitious.

This chapter includes a brief overview of a relatively new weight loss technique: the use of temperature. The main idea is that your body is required to maintain a core temperature of 98.6 degrees Fahrenheit regardless of your environment. So by exposing yourself to some degree of cold, you should be able to force your metabolism to expend more energy—and, therefore, burn fat. This is a bit like leaving all your windows in your home open in the winter: you'd probably get an unpleasant shock when your heating bill arrived.

One of the main proponents of temperature-based weight loss is NASA scientist Ray Cronise. Cronise was able to lose thirty pounds in six weeks while incorporating thermal techniques into his diet, and he argues that you can lose up to 50% more weight in half the time by consistently exposing yourself to lower temperatures.

Cronise initially became interested in thermal-based weight loss when he saw a TV program claiming that Olympic swimmer Michael Phelps consumes 12,000 calories per day. Now 12,000 calories is an incredible amount of food to eat in a single day. A "normal" person who requires about 2000 calories could gain nearly three pounds of fat (at 3500 calories per pound) in a single day on such a diet!

Cronise did a quick calculation and found that even Michael Phelps could not possibly burn that many extra calories through exercise alone. (Recall from the previous chapter that the human body is extremely efficient—even jogging only burns around 100 calories per mile). Cronise then came up with the theory that the difference must be accounted for by the thermal effect of Phelps being submerged in water for so many hours per day. Water is a very effective conductor and will rapidly pull heat from your body. This is why the victims of boating accidents at sea often have very short survival times.

Motivated by this insight, Cronise added thermal techniques to his weight loss plan. He turned down the thermostat in his home, wore fewer layers of clothing in cold weather and slept without blankets at night. The result was weight loss that occurred far more rapidly that he had previously experienced through diet alone. You can find out more at Ray Cronise's website, http://hypothermics.com and also in a 9-minute presentation he gave at the TED MED conference (to find the video, google "Ray Cronise TED").

Ray Cronise's work on thermal-based diets gained a lot of visibility with the publication of Tim Ferriss's book The Four-Hour Body, which includes a chapter focusing on temperature as a weight loss tool. Ferriss takes things a few steps further, offering up a theory about "brown" fat (as opposed to normal "white" fat) and how you can use extreme techniques such as ice baths to potentially burn even more fat.

Dr. Pierre Dukan is also a fan of thermal weight loss, and in his book he recommends wrapping up less in winter and taking cold showers. Both Dukan and Cronise advocate drinking cold water. Dukan even provides precise numbers, suggesting that taking a cold shower for two minutes can burn 100 calories, and that drinking two quarts of refrigerated water burns 60 calories—enough to expend 22,000 calories (or six pounds of fat) over the course of a year.

So what should we make of all this? Can you really lose lots of weight just by staying cold? While the case that advocates like Ray Cronise make seems to hold up logically, there has so far not been a great deal of research that strongly supports thermal weight loss.

The one formal research study I found really does not offer especially exciting results. In a 2007 project at Maastricht University in the Netherlands, scientists conducted an experiment on 11 healthy male subjects. The men spent two sessions in a temperature-controlled chamber: one session at normal room temperature, and a second at a cold temperature, but not cold enough to cause shivering. The men spent 82 hours (or about 3.5 24-hour days) exposed to cold. The scientists then compared the amount of energy expended (calories burned) by the men during the two sessions.

The results? The men did indeed expend more energy in the cold environment. The researchers measured a difference of 0.32 millijoules per day—or about 76 calories per day. Keep in mind that to get those 76 calories the men were kept in the cold chamber for an entire 24 hours. Since a pound of fat is equivalent to 3500 calories, if these results are accurate, you would need to stay in the cold chamber for 46 days (and nights) to lose one pound.

So one the one hand we have a formal study that says staying cold for a full 24 hours expends 76 calories. On the other hand, we have Dr. Dukan claiming that a two-minute cold shower burns 100 calories, and drinking two liters of cold water burns 60! Even allowing for the fact that water is a more effective conductor of heat than air, that is a pretty big disconnect. Clearly any precise numbers offered up by those advocating thermal weight loss techniques should be taken with a healthy degree of skepticism.

So far, the argument for temperature-based fat loss seems to be largely anecdotal and not well supported by evidence. Even the story of Michael Phelps eating 12,000 calories a day raises some obvious questions. Apparently, this number came from a TV program, but has it really been verified? If Ray Cronise's theory about the thermal effect of exposure to water is correct, then it can't work only for Michael Phelps: shouldn't all serious swimmers who spend hours every day in the pool need to eat enormous amounts of food? Surely there are a lot of competitive swimmers at the college and even the high school level who practice a great deal; I find it a bit difficult to believe that swimmers find it necessary to eat so much more than athletes who engage in non-water sports.

MY RECOMMENDATIONS

While I tend to be skeptical of many of the specific claims made for thermal weight loss, I believe that it can be a useful way to augment your diet, and I have used it myself, primarily while walking in cooler temperatures. Here are my recommendations:

- Drinking cold water every day is easy and costs you nothing, so I would certainly suggest trying this idea. Remember that on any protein-intensive diet, it is critical to drink plenty of water. So why not make it cold water?

- You can combine cold exposure with walking by dressing in layers and then removing one or more layers during your walk. I often use this technique. For safety, always carry sufficient warm clothes with you and take care to keep your extremities (hands, ears, etc.) warm. This is not something you want to attempt in truly cold weather, but it works well in spring or fall.

- In general, for cold exposure to be effective I suspect it needs to be done on a long-term, consistent basis. Turning down your home thermostat may be a reasonable idea—especially if you can justify this through other means as well (a lower heating bill, less carbon in the air, etc.). Obviously, this is something that you would need to negotiate with any other members of your household.

- I would not recommend short-term, extreme techniques like ice baths and cold showers (unless this is something you enjoy). These ideas sound gimmicky to me, and the results from the study conducted in the Netherlands make it difficult to believe that any benefit from such a brief exposure would be worth the misery you are inflicting on yourself.

CONCLUSION

In this book, have tried to clearly and concisely convey virtually everything I have learned in my twenty-year battle against weight gain. The information has come from a combination of personal experience and experimentation, as well as extensive research.

I am a strong believer in using any effective technique I can find in my efforts to stay healthy, and I don't hesitate to recommend modern innovations like high quality protein powder and green supplement powder. There is no doubt that innovations in food processing—and especially the advent of packaged and fast foods—has a lot to do with the fact that two thirds of Americans are now overweight or obese. However, given the demands of daily life, for most people, it is simply not realistic to try to turn back the clock and eat a diet consisting entirely of healthy, non-processed whole foods. Losing weight and keeping it off is not easy, and I think you should feel free to use every tool in the toolbox to make it happen.

Here is a very brief summary of some of the most critical ideas I've tried to cover:

- Protein is the most critical macronutrient. Consuming more protein while limiting carbohydrates will help you lose fat and maintain muscle.

- For rapid weight loss, use high quality protein drinks that also include the phytochemicals found in green vegetables to replace one or two meals a day.
- Keep the ingredients for protein drinks handy at home, in the office and/or in your car so you'll never have an excuse to resort to fast food or processed snack foods.
- Once you achieve your weight loss goal, calculate a "line in the sand" and have a strategy in place for when you cross that line. Don't kid yourself: virtually everyone starts to re-gain weight at some point. Be ready for it, and don't let things get out of hand.
- Try to incorporate exercise, including both walking and, if possible, weight training into your lifestyle. This will accelerate your fat loss and help you maintain your muscle mass as well as achieve cardiovascular fitness.
- Thermal weight loss techniques are worth looking at as a supplemental strategy, but much more research needs to be done in this area.

Whether you choose to follow the specific weight loss plan I have laid out in this book or use the protein drinks and other techniques in conjunction with another diet, I believe you will find that the ideas I have presented here really work. I can say with honesty that these techniques changed my life dramatically for the better—and I hope and expect that the same will be true for you.

CONTACTING THE AUTHOR

Comments, suggestions and corrections can be sent to the author by email at: proexpdiet@yahoo.com.

More information is also available on the book's website: http://www.ProteinExpressDiet.com.

9158895R00064

Made in the USA
San Bernardino, CA
06 March 2014